Chronic Fatigue Syndrome

a natural way to treat M.E.

Chronic Fatigue Syndrome

a natural way to treat M.E.

Professor Basant K. Puri

MA (Cantab), PhD, MB, BChir, BSc (Hons)
MathSci, MRCPsych, DipStat, MMath

Consultant/Professor, MRI Unit, Imaging
Sciences Department, MRC Clinical Sciences
Centre, Hammersmith Hospital, London, UK
and Head of the Lipid Neuroscience Group,
Imperial College, London, UK

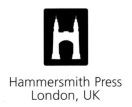

Hammersmith Press
London, UK

First published in 2005 by Hammersmith Press Limited,
496 Fulham Palace Road, London SW6 6JD, UK

© Hammersmith Press Limited 2005
Reprinted 2005
Revised reprint 2006
Third reprint 2006
Fourth reprint 2007

British Library Cataloguing in Publication Data: A CIP record for this book is available from
the British Library.

ISBN 1-905140-00-2   ISBN 978-1-905140-00-8

Designed by Julie Bennett, Bespoke Publishing Ltd.
Printed and bound in Great Britain by TJ International Ltd.

Contents

1. A breakthrough   7

2. What is chronic fatigue syndrome?   10

3. All in the mind?   22

4. How and why fatty acids can help   46

5. How to take fatty acids   74

6. The vitamin and mineral cofactors   84

7. Other benefits from taking fatty acids   97

8. Treating chronic fatigue syndrome naturally   108

    Glossary   128

    References   136

    Further sources of information   142

    Useful names and addresses   144

    Index   147

1

A breakthrough

In July 2004 I received the following letter:

16 July 2004
Dr Basant Puri
MRI Dept.
Hammersmith Hospital

Dear Dr Puri

As you requested, I write to report on my husband's condition after taking 7 VegEPA capsules per day for three months.

[He] was diagnosed with very severe ME 6 years ago and sadly had to take very early retirement at age 49.

After 3 months on 7 capsules per day, we are thrilled to report that [he] can now actually read a book – something totally beyond him for all these years! It would appear that his memory and brain 'fog' have improved and [he] is excited about this.

He is a very intelligent man ...

May I take this opportunity, Dr Puri, to convey to you our heartfelt thanks and appreciation. We are truly grateful.

Yours sincerely

If this were a one-off positive response to the natural treatment I use in chronic fatigue syndrome or M.E., then no one would be too surprised. After all, the placebo effect, whereby a patient can improve simply by seeing a doctor even if given 'dummy' pills, is well known. This letter, however, is far from unique.

In this book I shall describe why, early in this new millennium, I came to the conclusion that one of the key components needed to treat chronic fatigue syndrome is a combination of ultra-pure EPA (free of any DHA) and virgin evening primrose oil. (You will read all about EPA and DHA – what they mean and how to obtain them – in Chapters 4 and 5.) The first product available to the general public that contains just this very combination, of ultra-pure EPA (free of any DHA) and virgin evening primrose oil, became available in April 2004. This is when I started treating my chronic fatigue syndrome patients with this natural product, known as VegEPA. Starting just one-month later, unsolicited reports started coming in to the company which manufactures VegEPA praising the product and its marvellous benefits. Within three months, as I started to see my patients at their three-month follow-up appointments, I was able to verify that striking clinical improvements were occurring in most of them. To date, over 80% of my patients have improved within three months, no matter for how long they have suffered from this dreadful debilitating disease previously.

I have written this book to share the rationale for this natural treatment, and the findings to date, with open-minded individuals. Whether you are a sufferer, a friend, or a relative of a patient who has witnessed at first hand how cruel this illness can be, a medical practitioner, a dietician, or a practitioner of complementary medicine or nutritional therapy, you should find this book of great interest.

The observant reader will have noticed that I talk about chronic fatigue syndrome as being a disease or illness. I believe that it is indeed a genuine physical illness, with clinical features over which patients have little or no control. In the next chapter I shall describe the main symptoms and signs of chronic fatigue syndrome or M.E. My stance on the disease is somewhat contentious, and reflects the controversy that has surrounded the nature of this condition in academic medical circles. A major spur to this debate occurred in 1970. Two psychiatrists published a paper in the *British Medical Journal*, in which they claimed retrospectively that a large outbreak of what I consider to have been chronic fatigue syndrome/M.E. was caused by 'mass hysteria' (McEvedy and Beard, 1970). This outbreak occurred in 1955 in The Royal Free Hospital, a teaching hospital in London, England. (You can find the full references in one of the appendices at the end of this book. The first part of each reference in this appendix gives the surnames and initials of the authors of key medical and scientific papers, book chapters and books that are mentioned in this book. These are followed by the year of publication and then the title of the work. Finally, for medical and scientific journals, the title of the journal is given, together with the journal volume number and the page numbers within that volume. For book chapters and books, the name of the publisher is given. In the text of this book, I shall refer to papers, chapters and books by giving the surnames of the authors and the year of publication.)

From then on, many psychiatrists have been prone to consider patients with chronic fatigue syndrome or M.E. as suffering from an hysterical or 'psychosomatic' illness. I shall have more to say in Chapter 3 about why I think chronic fatigue syndrome or M.E. is a real physical disease and not simply a condition that is 'all in the mind'. Meanwhile, in what may be a first in modern publishing history, I am happy to exclude from the intended readership of this book those leading academics, particularly in psychiatry, who claim that chronic fatigue syndrome or M.E. is largely psychosomatic; usually, authors go out of their way to encourage as many sales of their books as possible.

In the next chapter we shall look at the different names given to this condition. In general, I shall use the term 'chronic fatigue syndrome'. This should be taken as being synonymous with M.E.

2

What is chronic fatigue syndrome?

A brief history

Neurasthenia

The term 'neurasthenia' was introduced in the nineteenth century to describe a disease of the nervous system in which there was 'enfeeblement of the nervous force, which may have all degrees of severity, from slight loosening of these forces down to profound and general prostration' (Deale & Adams, 1894). The term was used to refer to a slightly nebulous disorder of mental functioning characterized by the occurrence of:

- General lassitude

- Irritability

- Difficulty with concentrating

- Worry

- Hypochondria.

These features are similar to those suffered by people with chronic fatigue syndrome.

A number of famous people were thought to have suffered from neurasthenia, raising the possibility that if alive today they would be diagnosed as suffering from chronic fatigue syndrome. One likely sufferer was the English poet Elizabeth Barrett Browning, who lived from 1806 to 1861. Following the death of her brother in a boating accident, she was said to have developed a nervous disorder that confined her to 'the sickroom' for many years. Another was the French novelist Marcel Proust, who lived from 1871 to 1922. He was a 'semi-invalid' all his life and at the age of 34, on his mother's death, withdrew completely from society.

There is some controversy as to whether or not the English nurse and founder of modern nursing, Florence Nightingale, suffered from chronic fatigue syndrome. Certainly she lived as an invalid in London from 1857 to 1880, although she was able to receive many visitors while lying on her couch. After her death, the general medical opinion was that she had suffered from neurasthenia. However, an article in the *British Medical Journal* by Young in 1995 concluded that she might, in fact, have been suffering from the infection chronic brucellosis having contracted acute brucellosis in the Crimea in 1854. This is a bacterial infection, also known as Malta fever, Mediterranean fever or undulant fever, which was named after Dr David Bruce, a British Army medical doctor who isolated the causative microbes only in 1887.

Even if Florence Nightingale did indeed have chronic brucellosis her condition might still have been diagnosed as chronic fatigue syndrome had the term been in use at the time, according to Dr. Robert Fekety of the University of Michigan Medical Center. Dr Fekety wrote:

> The evidence strongly supports the concept that brucellar infection was the 'cause' of ... chronic brucellosis, and that it would now be called the chronic fatigue syndrome. (Fekety, 1994; page 113.)

The concept of chronic fatigue syndrome or M.E. developed from the disorder known as neurasthenia. In many ways, the history of this development reflects a fundamental dichotomy between the medical disciplines of neurology and psychiatry and the turf war that is continually fought within the medical profession.

On the one hand, nervous system symptoms and signs are attributed to physical or 'organic' lesions (pathology) by neurologists.

Symptoms are the features of a condition that are experienced by the patient, whereas signs are those features that are elicited from the patient, usually by a doctor during a physical examination. Thus, if a patient reports feeling fatigue, then this is a symptom (said to be 'subjective'), while if I observe that my patient looks clinically anaemic when I examine them, then that is a sign elicited by me.

On the other hand, psychiatry traditionally deals with conditions that are not considered to have a clear organic cause. The trouble with this duality is that the vast majority of scientists now believe that all mental phenomena must ultimately have a physical basis. This means that all 'psychiatric' symptoms, such as feeling depressed, must have some organic explanation (or at the least, some abnormality in the 'software' of the brain).

The condition described by the term neurasthenia eventually evolved into what we now know as chronic fatigue syndrome. The template for the disagreement between those who consider that chronic fatigue syndrome has a physical basis (the 'neurology' side) and those who consider it to be psychosomatic (the 'psychiatry' side) was set right from the start, with a controversy as to who was the first actually to introduce the term neurasthenia in the nineteenth century.

On one side was Beard, a neurologist working in New York, who introduced the term neurasthenia in his landmark paper entitled 'Neurasthenia, or nervous exhaustion' in 1869 in the *Boston Medical and Surgical Journal*. George Beard argued that the nervous system could become exhausted by various physical and social demands made upon it. On the other side was Van Deusen, a psychiatrist working in Kalamazoo, who also introduced the term neurasthenia in 1869, in a paper entitled 'Observations of a form of nervous prostration, (neurasthenia), culminating in insanity', in the *American Journal of Insanity*.

During the first world war, neurasthenia was a relatively popular diagnosis, used for invaliding many soldiers out of the trenches in the European arena of warfare. However, as neurology established itself as a modern scientifically-grounded medical discipline, the diagnostic classification of neurasthenia gradually disappeared from it. In American psychiatry, this category is no longer in use at all in their current psychiatric classification system, the *Diagnostic and Statistical Manual of Mental Disorders, Fourth edition, Text Revision (DSM-IV-TR)*. In contrast, the World Health Organization still includes neurasthenia as a psychiatric disorder under its classification of 'neurotic' disorders in its current, tenth, revision of the International Classification of Diseases (ICD-10). (By neurotic disorders they mean a group of psychiatric conditions in which distressing symptoms occur which are alien to the person's personality. Examples include phobias and hypochondriasis.) *The ICD-10 Classification* gives the following description of neurasthenia:

Considerable cultural variations occur in the presentation of this disorder; two main types occur, with substantial overlap. In one type, the main feature is a complaint of increased fatigue after mental effort, often associated with some decrease in occupational performance or coping efficiency in daily tasks. The mental fatiguability is typically described as an unpleasant intrusion of distracting associations or recollections, difficulty in concentrating, and generally inefficient thinking. In the other type, the emphasis is on feelings of bodily or physical weakness and exhaustion after only minimal effort, accompanied by a feeling of muscular aches and pains and inability to relax. In both types, a variety of other unpleasant physical feelings, such as dizziness, tension headaches, and a sense of general instability, is common. Worry about decreasing mental and bodily well-being, irritability, anhedonia (a loss of the ability to enjoy activities that were previously found to be pleasurable), and varying minor degrees of both depression and anxiety are all common. Sleep is often disturbed in its initial and middle phases but hypersomnia may also be prominent.

Los Angeles County Hospital epidemic

In 1934 there was an outbreak of a chronic fatigue syndrome-type illness amongst the medical and nursing staff of the Los Angeles

County Hospital. Almost two hundred members of staff were affected, with symptoms such as myalgia (muscle pain), emotional distress, and emotional lability (rapid mood swings), and features, such as sensory symptoms, suggesting involvement of the nervous system outside the brain. At the time, there was concern that this epidemic might herald an outbreak of poliomyelitis. However, in spite of muscle weakness, the key features of poliomyelitis did not develop: muscle wasting did not feature, paralysis usually did not occur, and samples of the cerebrospinal fluid that bathes the brain and spinal cord (obtained via a 'spinal tap' or lumbar puncture) were not found to be abnormal.

Royal Free disease

Like the Los Angeles County Hospital epidemic, the episode at the Royal Free Hospital (a teaching hospital in London, UK) also affected nursing and medical staff. It took place in 1955. On 13th July of that year, a resident doctor and a ward sister were admitted as in-patients at the start of an epidemic that eventually affected almost three hundred members of staff. The commonest symptoms were: profound malaise, headache, low-grade fever, sore throat, nausea, severe depression, swings in emotional state, dizziness, vertigo, and neck-, back-, limb- and chest-pain. Signs included generalized enlargement of the lymph nodes, particularly those in the neck (cervical lymphadenopathy), and muscle changes such as 'fasciculation' (in which the muscles appear to show a rippling motion), spasm, twitching and tingling. In most patients there was clinical evidence that the brain and spinal cord were affected. About a quarter of the patients had problems with their urinary bladder. On physical examination, the liver was enlarged in about a tenth of the patients. In general, the illness became worse during the second and third weeks after clinical onset. Many patients continued to suffer for many years after this outbreak.

Sadly, some of the original victims of the Royal Free outbreak are still suffering from the effects of chronic fatigue syndrome at the time of writing. One of my patients told me in mid-

2004 of a lady in her seventies who lives in her part of north London and who has continued to suffer from chronic fatigue syndrome since 1955, when she caught the illness while working at the Royal Free Hospital.

In spite of the physical symptoms and signs just noted Dr Colin McEvedy and Dr Alfred William Beard, both psychiatrists, published a paper in the *British Medical Journal* in 1970 that drew a quite different conclusion. In this paper they re-assessed the symptoms and signs from which the Royal Free epidemic patients had suffered, classifying them mostly as 'subjective' and comparing them with those seen in a 'previous epidemic of overbreathing' at a girls' school, also described by Dr McEvedy (1966). On the basis of this reanalysis, Colin McEvedy and Bill Beard proposed that this Royal Free epidemic had, in fact, been a case of 'mass hysteria'. While the related leading article in that issue of the *British Medical Journal* complimented the authors 'for performing a valuable service in drawing attention to the possible psychological origins of some outbreaks of illness that are disseminated in an explosive manner' it also urged caution about 'the limitations of retrospective epidemiological inquiry; much of the positive psychiatric evidence required for a conclusive judgement on the nature of [these] epidemics is inevitably lacking.' Nevertheless, this paper has turned out to be very influential.

Mass hysteria is also known as epidemic hysteria or communicable hysteria. Dr Christopher Freeman, a consultant psychotherapist based at the Royal Edinburgh Hospital, published the following account of its features in 1998.

[Outbreaks of epidemic hysteria] have a number of common features: they tend to occur in women, often schoolgirls; they usually arise in an atmosphere of stress or constraint such as a boarding school or other institution; they frequently begin in an individual of high status, with a peer group then developing the same symptoms, which thereafter spread down the status hierarchy, and from older to younger. New cases appear at times of social contact rather than during classes and those who initially deal with the outbreak are often indecisive and anxious.

Possibly in anticipation of the negative reaction that their conclusion might give rise to in some quarters, Drs Colin McEvedy and Bill Beard stated:

Many people will feel that the diagnosis of hysteria is distasteful. This ought not to prevent its discussion, but perhaps makes it worthwhile to point out that the diagnosis of hysteria is not a slur on either the individuals or the institution involved.

Unfortunately, despite the caution urged in the related leading article, this 1970 paper marked the beginning of the view by psychiatry in general that chronic fatigue syndrome is essentially psychosomatic in nature.

Revised CDC criteria of Fukuda and colleagues

In general, the criteria used by doctors when making a diagnosis clinically are not as strict as those used when carrying out a research project. For a research project it is important to make the patient group that is being studied as uniform as possible in terms of their symptoms and signs.

The criteria for diagnosing chronic fatigue syndrome or M.E. that my colleagues and I tend to use in our research into this area are a revision of the original American criteria issued by the CDC (Centers for Disease Control and Prevention) in Atlanta, Georgia. These revised criteria were published in the *Annals of Internal Medicine* in December 1994 (Fukuda and colleagues, 1994). The authors were from a number of international centres of excellence (including the CDC) and included the eminent individuals listed in the box.

**Authors of CDC criteria for diagnosing
chronic fatigue syndrome**

Keiji Fukuda, MD, MPH, from the Division of Viral and
Rickettsial Diseases, National Center for Infectious
Diseases, Centers for Disease Control and Prevention,
Atlanta, Georgia;

Stephen E. Straus, MD, from the Laboratory of Clinical
Investigation and Division of Microbiology and Infectious
Diseases, National Institute of Allergy and Infectious
Diseases, National Institutes of Health, Bethesda,
Maryland;

Ian Hickie, MD, FRANZCP, from the School of Psychiatry,
Prince Henry Hospital, University of New South Wales,
Sydney, Australia;

Michael C. Sharpe, MRCP, MRCPsych, from the University
of Oxford Department of Psychiatry, Warneford Hospital,
Oxford, United Kingdom; and

Anthony L. Komaroff, MD, FACP of Harvard University,
Boston, Massachusetts.

(Other authors included James G. Dobbins, PhD, and the
International Chronic Fatigue Syndrome Study Group.)

A summary of the criteria for diagnosing chronic fatigue
syndrome put together by this prestigious line-up, drawn from
amongst the world's leading researchers, is as follows.

1. Exclude any other cause for chronic fatigue.
2. Self-reported persistent or relapsing fatigue for six or more
   consecutive months.
3. Four or more of the following symptoms are concurrently

present for over six months:
    i. Impaired memory or concentration
    ii. Sore throat
    iii. Tender cervical (neck) or axillary (armpit) lymph nodes
    iv. Muscle pain
    v. Multi-joint pain
    vi. New headaches
    vii. Unrefreshing sleep
    viii. Post-exertion malaise.

Within this framework, self-reported, persistent fatigue of one month or longer is defined as being prolonged fatigue, and only becomes chronic fatigue after it has lasted for at least six consecutive months. This criterion relating to the length of time the illness has lasted certainly helps in standardizing the disease for research purposes. However, in clinical practice I do not require patients to have suffered from the illness for at least six months before I am prepared to make this diagnosis. I do, however, find criteria numbers 1 and 3 in the above list helpful.

The name of the disease

A number of different names have been given to what would appear to be essentially the same cluster of symptoms and signs, or at least highly overlapping clusters.

The term neurasthenia, introduced in 1869, has been considered earlier in this chapter. One of the disadvantages of the name neurasthenia is that it is associated with a primarily psychiatric disorder, being, as mentioned earlier, in the current *ICD-10 Classification of Mental and Behavioural Disorders*.

M.E., standing for myalgic encephalomyelitis, was introduced in an editorial in the *Lancet* in May 1956. The first part of this name, myalgic, refers to the clinical features that may occur in the muscles, for instance muscle fatigue, pain, fasciculation (in which there are fine movements of small regions of muscles), spasm, twitching or tingling. The second part of the name, encephalomyelitis, refers to inflammation of the brain and spinal cord; to date, there is no convincing evidence that such inflammation is a characteristic feature of this condition.

Post-viral fatigue syndrome, or PVFS, was introduced in the 1980s and is a testament to how commonly the disorder appears to develop after a viral-like infection. A difficulty with this name is that it does not take into account those cases of the disorder in which there is no clear evidence of development following a viral infection.

The term chronic fatigue and immune dysfunction syndrome, or CFIDS, is particularly common in the United States of America, where it is favoured by many patients' organizations and self-help groups.

In this book, the terms chronic fatigue syndrome and M.E. are favoured. However, even the name 'chronic fatigue syndrome' has disadvantages, such as the implication that one cannot be suffering from the disorder unless there is fatigue that is long-lasting.

How common is it?

Estimates of how common chronic fatigue syndrome is in the general population vary enormously. This is hardly surprising, given the controversy that exists in relation to the cause of the disorder (organic or psychosomatic) and the differing names and diagnostic criteria that can be applied. In spite of earlier suggestions that it might mainly affect women ('mass hysteria') or young, upwardly mobile people ('yuppie 'flu'), chronic fatigue syndrome appears not to recognize any barriers of sex, class or ethnicity.

The symptom of fatigue alone is very common. Between March and September 2000, in the United Kingdom, over 8,800 individuals aged between 16 and 24 years and living in private households in England, Wales and Scotland (including the Highlands and Islands) were interviewed as part of a national survey. This was carried out by the Social Survey Division of the Office for National Statistics on behalf of the Department of Health, the Scottish Executive and the

National Assembly for Wales. The results of this large survey were published as *Psychiatric Morbidity among Adults living in Private Households, 2000* by Nicola Singleton and colleagues, and showed that, during the week before the interview, 32% of women and 23% of men had suffered from fatigue. Taking both genders together, overall 27% of all the adults interviewed had suffered from fatigue during that week. In fact, the only symptom that occurred more commonly during that week was sleep problems, which were reported by 34% of the women and 24% of the men (29% overall).

As for chronic fatigue syndrome itself, the published figures for how common it is vary widely. As I have already said, this is not surprising, in view of the different criteria that have been used to identify cases, not to mention the difficulty that some doctors have had in agreeing that the disease exists in the first place.

Drs Niloofar Afari and Dedra Buchwald, from the Departments of Psychiatry and Behavioral Sciences and Medicine, University of Washington, Seattle, carried out a review of previous studies. This was published in the *American Journal of Psychiatry* in 2003. They found that, overall, up to 3% of the adult population suffer from chronic fatigue syndrome as defined by rigorous criteria such as the revised CDC criteria given earlier. Even higher are the rates of occurrence of disabling fatigue that does not meet strict diagnostic criteria.

Figures for chronic fatigue syndrome in adolescents have also been obtained. These are generally lower than the maximum figures obtained for adults. In 2004, the National Jewish Medical and Research Center in Denver, Colorado, published the results of a study of chronic fatigue syndrome in adolescents aged between 12 and 17 years based on a random sampling of the residents of Wichita, Kansas (Jones and colleagues, 2004). The adults identified by these means in turn gave the researchers details of any adolescents lived in their households, and, further, details of any who suffered from fatigue. Selected adolescents were then invited to a clinic for the purpose of diagnosis. Those adolescents with fatigue were followed-up annually for three years by telephone interview and clinical evaluation. Overall, 8,586 adolescents were identified. Of these, 138 had fatigue for a period of at least one month, and most of these 138 (107 or 78%) had chronic fatigue (defined as having lasted for at least six months) at some time during the three-year follow-up. So, during the three-year period, 1.6% of the adolescents had an M.E.-like illness (which did not necessarily meet the CDC criterion of lasting for at least 6 months), while just over 1.2% had chronic fatigue.

In another study of chronic fatigue syndrome in children and adolescents, also published in 2004, Professor Anne Farmer from the Institute of Psychiatry in London, together with former colleagues from the Department of Psychological Medicine of the University of Wales College of Medicine in Cardiff, Wales, looked at how common this condition is in 8- to 17-year olds. There were two parts to this study. First, parents of twins (from two 'twin series') were asked to complete questionnaires that enquired about whether either or both of their twins had suffered from more than a few days of disabling fatigue. The second part of the study consisted of carrying out telephone interviews with the children who had experienced such a level of fatigue. Overall, 2.3% of the children had experienced disabling fatigue lasting at least three months, while the corresponding figure was 1.3% for those who had suffered symptoms that met the 1994 revised CDC criteria of Fukuda and colleagues.

So, for a country with a population the size of the United Kingdom's, there may be between 750,000 and 1,500,000 sufferers of chronic fatigue syndrome or an illness that almost reaches the current diagnostic criteria. This is a huge number. Even using the figures from studies that have given smaller rates of occurrence, the numbers are still large; in 2002, the BBC online web site was quoting a figure of 243,000 sufferers in the United Kingdom. The corresponding figures for the United States are, of course, even higher, and might range from 1,500,000 to an astonishing 9,000,000 sufferers.

3

All in the mind?

In the previous two chapters we have seen how, beginning with the 1970 *British Medical Journal* article of the two psychiatrists, McEvedy and Beard, the notion has grown within the medical profession, and particularly within psychiatry, that the Royal Free epidemic of 1955 and other afflictions of chronic fatigue syndrome-like illness actually represent cases of 'psychosomatic' disorders. In this chapter we shall see that there is a great deal of evidence that indicates that patients suffering from the clinical features that occurred during the Royal Free epidemic are likely to be suffering from a physical (organic) illness, rather than from an hysterical disorder (as suggested by McEvedy and Beard). This evidence comes from a consideration of viral infections, changes in the immune system, blood fatty acid levels, and brain biochemistry.

Viral infections

As a clinician, I cannot help but notice that most of my M.E. patients give me a clear history of having suffered from a viral infection-like illness just before coming down with chronic fatigue syndrome. The association can be very clear when witnessed by a parent.

Take my patient Mary (not her real name), for example. Mary is a 20-year-old student at a university in England who has struggled with chronic fatigue syndrome ever since the age of 12 years, when it was diagnosed by a consultant physician. Mary's mother has given me a detailed history of her daughter's illness. After suffering from numerous episodes of ear infections as a child, Mary came down with an influenza-like illness at the age of 12. This lasted five to six days. After making a partial recovery, Mary again appeared to catch a similar illness a few weeks later. This time, Mary was laid low by the illness, and she has never seemed to recover fully. Both Mary and her mother can mark the start of profound fatigue, muscle pain and weakness, and poor concentration to the second episode of the influenza-like illness at the age of 12.

Another example is given by my patient Christopher. He is a 45-year-old married man who has been suffering from chronic fatigue syndrome for 12 years. Prior to the onset of the illness, he was a very driven, hard working, highly successful businessman. Then he came down with an influenza-like illness. 'I was laid low by the 'flu for a week, Dr Puri', he recalled. 'I was utterly exhausted and just couldn't move. It was so unlike me.' Following the apparent 'resolution' of the viral-like illness, Christopher found he was suffering from symptoms of chronic fatigue syndrome, and until seeing me, had never been able to resume work again. Sadly, his company collapsed. However, fortunately for him, his wife fully believed that he was suffering from a genuine illness, and she has stayed with him and done her best to help him.

Once an acute viral illness appears to be over, this does not necessarily imply that the causative virus has disappeared from the body. On the contrary, it is perfectly possible for such a virus to establish itself in the body at a sub-clinical level; the virus might still be present and causing a persistent infection, but the acute symptoms and signs may no longer be evident. Chicken pox is a particularly well-known example; after infection the virus that causes it can lie dormant for years and then manifest itself as 'shingles' when triggered by other health problems.

Viruses are able to fuse their cell membranes with those of the host (human) cells that they are invading. Once complete fusion is achieved, the viral contents, including viral genetic information (in the form of DNA or RNA), can readily be passed into the host cell. The infected cell is not necessarily killed; it can be parasitized by the virus so that it remains alive but its functions are altered to suit the virus. We shall see in the next chapter that one of the effects of many viral species is that they can prevent cells from producing important omega-3 and omega-6 fatty acids such as the omega-3 fatty acid EPA (eicosapentaenoic acid). Such a strategy has advantages for a virus that is trying to establish itself in the human host, without killing off the host completely. A key advantage for the virus, described more fully in Chapter 4, is related to the fact that EPA is directly and indirectly lethal to many viruses.

There are many features of chronic fatigue syndrome that are consistent with it being caused by an infectious agent such as a virus. For example, epidemics have occurred of the disease that could have been the result of person-to-person spread, as in the cases of the Los Angeles County Hospital epidemic of 1934 and the Royal Free Hospital epidemic of 1955. Again, those affected in such epidemics are often those most likely to be exposed to an infectious agent – doctors and nurses, in particular. There is also the common occurrence of a history of a viral-like illness just before the onset of chronic fatigue syndrome. Some of the features of chronic fatigue syndrome, such as the chronic fatiguing illness itself and the muscle weakness, are known sequelae of viral infections.

So, an infectious agent is a strong possibility. However, even if there is an infectious agent that is causing most cases of chronic fatigue syndrome, we should not assume that it is necessarily a virus. Towards the end of the First World War, there was a worldwide influenza pandemic of horrific proportions that killed many millions of people. Starting in 1917, some of the survivors of this pandemic who had not apparently caught the infection themselves were found to be suffering from a terrible condition in which they became essentially mute and hardly able to move, as if they were living statues. (The condition often started with headaches, malaise, lethargy, insomnia and strange movements of the eyes.) Most of those affected by this condition, known as encephalitis lethargica or von Economo encephalitis, were institutionalized for life; some of the long-term sufferers in an institution in New York were brilliantly described by Dr Oliver Sacks in his book *Awakenings*.

Given the coincidence with the influenza pandemic, it was naturally assumed by some researchers that if encephalitis lethargica were a genuine neurological illness (rather than a psychosomatic or hysterical disorder) then the cause might be a virus; there were certainly features of the condition that pointed to an infectious agent. To date, no evidence has been found of the genetic material of any influenza virus or indeed any virus at all in the post mortem (autopsy) brains of affected patients. Since the end of the First World War, more cases of encephalitis lethargica have occurred, right up to the present day, although it is now far less common than it was just after the influenza pandemic of the First World War. In 2004, Dr Russell Dale, working at the Institute of Child Health at Great Ormond Street Hospital, London, published a paper in the journal *Brain* in which he and his colleagues showed that there was evidence that more recent cases of encephalitis lethargica had been infected not by a virus but by a bacterium, namely the *Streptococcus*. In fact, most patients with the illness have a clinical history of having suffered from a (Streptococcal) sore throat before the onset of the disease.

So far as chronic fatigue syndrome or M.E. is concerned, there are two messages I wish to draw from this potted history of encephalitis lethargica. First, the infectious agent responsible for chronic fatigue syndrome may not necessarily be a virus. Second, even with all the tools of modern medical research at its disposal, it has taken 87 years (from 1917 to 2004) to identify a likely causative agent in the case of encephalitis lethargica; we should be patient, therefore, if an infectious agent has not yet been identified in the case of chronic fatigue syndrome. (It is tempting to draw a third message, relating to the fact that in the 1920s and 1930s some psychiatrists interpreted some of the features of encephalitis lethargica in psychodynamic terms. In other words, those psychiatrists thought that there was nothing physically wrong with these patients. Instead, the patients were suffering from an illness that was all in the mind.)

Incidentally, some readers might be wondering if there is any evidence that chronic fatigue syndrome may also be related to a bacterial infection such as that associated with a Streptococcal sore throat. From my clinical experience, I suspect that the answer is negative. My patient Mary, for example, has been treated with various powerful antibiotics for most of her life. In fact, when she was first seen by me, she had been taking antibiotics (prescribed by her previous doctor) continuously for several years. If a bacterial infection was present, it should have been killed off by the antibiotics many years before, and yet Mary continued to suffer from full-blown chronic fatigue syndrome.

Changes in the immune system

Our bodies are endowed with special cells, such as the white blood cells that circulate through our arteries and veins, and chemicals, such as antibodies, which together constitute the immune system and which mediate our defence against invasion by foreign bodies such as viruses and unfriendly bacteria. These micro-organisms, and others such as fungi and protozoa (single-celled animal cells such as Amoebae), are able to cause disease. In fact, if they are allowed to multiply unabated, they can eventually take over the host body and cause its death.

External barriers to infection

The first barrier against potentially infectious micro-organisms lies with the defences that our bodies have at regions that may be directly exposed to contact with the external environment. Our skin, when intact, presents a physical barrier to these organisms. Fatty acids and certain relatively harmless micro-organisms that live on our skin also help protect us from more dangerous organisms.

We expose the main tubing of our lungs to potentially infectious micro-organisms every time we breathe in. Our defences here include sticky mucus in the bronchial passages, in which micro-organisms can become stuck. There are cells lining these passages that have little hair-like projections (the cilia) which waft the mucus up and out of the lungs. In fact, even before the air gets to the lungs, some particles are removed by the rapid movement of the air over the turbinate bones of the nasal passages.

Micro-organisms can also enter the body in the food we eat and the fluids we drink, not to mention children sucking on dirty objects and then swallowing the organisms on them. All of these enter lower parts of the gut, which can be thought of as a continuous 'tube' open at both ends. (One end is at the mouth. The other is at the anus.) Part of our defences includes the highly acidic nature of the contents of the stomach, which can kill many micro-organisms, or at least slow down their ability to multiply. Any organism that survives this then has to deal with a sudden and large change in acidity to the much more alkaline environment of the small intestine. If this, too, is survived, then the micro-organisms have to compete with friendly organisms (such as friendly bacteria or 'commensals') that live in the healthy large bowel. If the diet is rich in fibre, the unfriendly micro-organisms do not have much time to lurk in the intestines, as the call of nature rapidly forces the contents out through the other end of the gut.

Another opening to the outside world is provided by the vagina. Here, the body uses a combination of an acidic environment and the presence of friendly micro-organisms to act as a defence.

The tube through which urine passes (the urethra) is also a potential gateway into the body. Here, the passage of urine acts as a defence, by flushing out any potentially nasty organisms.

If any of these details have brought tears to your eyes, then this might be a good thing. The eyes are a potential way into the body, and tears and other secretions contain a strong enzyme (called lysozyme) that helps act as a defence.

In spite of these mechanisms, some potentially dangerous micro-organisms can and do break through our first line of defence. This may happen for a variety of reasons. There may be a breach in the defences caused by injury or inflammation, for example after an accident. Or there may be prolonged exchange of saliva with someone who has a viral infection. (As a medical student, I remember being taught that a good way of transmitting glandular fever (caused by the Epstein-Barr virus) is through 'deep kissing'. None of my textbooks gave further details, and none of my tutors ever bothered explaining the meaning of this term to me; to this day this remains an area of ignorance.) Direct transfer into the bloodstream is clearly a way of bypassing the first line of defences and getting micro-organisms directly into the blood. This can occur through blood transfusions with infected blood or blood products; through the use of contaminated (shared) needles by drug addicts and those being tattooed; through ano-rectal intercourse, when the anal sphincter might break and bleed, for example; and during first heterosexual intercourse, if there is rupture of the hymen. Sexual intercourse generally (both heterosexual and more especially male homosexual) can allow a wide variety of dangerous pathogens to be transmitted from an infected person into a previously uninfected person.

Lymphocytes

Whatever the cause, once the first line of defences has been breached, various types of immune responses can come into play. The exact nature of these depends to some extent on the type of infectious micro-organism and on the site of the infection itself. Some pathogens, such as viruses and some bacteria, actually invade our cells and reproduce inside them. In such cases, our immune system needs to be able to identify those of our cells that are infected and then act to destroy these (and therefore also the invading micro-organism inside them). The immune system acts in a different way to try to get rid of those pathogens that do not directly invade our cells but instead live in places such as the bloodstream and other fluids.

The immune system is extremely complex. For our purposes, we only need to look briefly at those parts of this system that appear to be of importance in chronic fatigue syndrome. In fact, we can narrow our consideration of the immune system down to just one group of cells, namely the lymphocytes. Lymphocytes are a particular type of white blood cell. It is easiest to think of lymphocytes as being divided into the following three types:

- B cells

- T cells

- Large granular lymphocytes (NK cells).

B cells produce antibodies that home in on specific targets. B cells are good at defending us from pathogens that are outside our cells, for example in the bloodstream.

T cells come in various types. Th1 cells are type-1 helper cells. They help other, Amoeba-like, white blood cells to engulf and destroy pathogens. Th2 cells are type-2 helper cells. They help B cells to reproduce and to make antibodies. Tc cells are T-cytotoxic cells. They destroy infected cells.

The large granular lymphocytes recognize cells that have become infected by viruses and also tumour cells. The large granular lymphocytes go on to damage such cells. This is known as natural killer cell activity, or NK cell activity for short.

Changes in lymphocytes in chronic fatigue syndrome

There have been many studies of changes in the immune system in chronic fatigue syndrome. Some of these are contradictory, and sometimes this is the result of poorly conducted studies. Difficulties abound, for example with respect to the way in which chronic fatigue syndrome/M.E. has been diagnosed in some investigations. Nevertheless, even after removing the more suspect reports, there remains a kernel of well-conducted robust observations. These relate to changes in:

• NK cell activity

• Th2 cell activity

• Tc cell activity.

There are many reports of a reduction in natural killer (NK) cell activity in chronic fatigue syndrome. For the interested reader, examples of good studies include those of: Caligiuri and colleagues published in 1987; Klimas and colleagues published in 1990; and Tirelli and colleagues published in 1993. (The full references appear at the back of this book.)

Well-conducted studies in chronic fatigue syndrome have also pointed to reduced Th1 cell activity in favour of a bias towards increased Th2 cell activity. One of these studies was that by Klimas and colleagues published in 1990 just mentioned. Two more recent studies that also favour this finding are those of: Visser and colleagues published in 1998; and Skowera and colleagues published in 2004.

The last of these studies, that by Skowera and colleagues (published in 2004) found a particular type of increased of Tc cell activity.

What do the lymphocyte changes mean?

The pattern of findings in chronic fatigue syndrome that has just been outlined, in which there is a bias away from Th1 cell activity towards Th2 cell activity, corresponds to what is known as a type 2 immune response. The reduction in natural killer (NK) cell activity in chronic fatigue syndrome is also consistent with a type 2 response, because NK cells help generate a Th1 response, and so reduced NK cell activity would favour a bias towards a Th2 or type 2 response.

There are several theories as to the implications of a type 2 response. For instance, a type 2 response could occur because the body is launching an immune response against its own normal (uninfected) cells – an autoimmune response. In fact, there is little consistent evidence to support the occurrence of an autoimmune response in chronic fatigue syndrome. Rather than rehearse all the other theories here, we may as well go straight to a model that fits the changes in lymphocyte function seen in this condition.

I think that the best explanation for the pattern of results seen in chronic fatigue syndrome, with reduced NK cell activity, reduced Th1 cell activity, increased Th2 cell activity and increased Tc cell activity, is that there is a pre-existing long-term viral infection, to which the immune system is reacting.

Blood fatty acid levels

Professor Peter Behan's group

In 1990, Professor Peter Behan (Professor of Neurology at the Institute of Neurological Sciences in Glasgow, Scotland), Professor Wilhelmina Behan (Professor of Muscle Pathology in Glasgow), and Professor David Horrobin (at that time Chief Executive Officer of Scotia Pharmaceuticals) published the results of a major study investigating fatty acids in chronic fatigue syndrome (or post-viral fatigue syndrome, as it was sometimes called at that time). Part of this study involved taking blood samples from each of 63 patients (27 men and 36 women) with chronic fatigue syndrome (postviral fatigue syndrome) and from 32 normal volunteers (20 men and 12 women) who were not suffering from any illnesses. The 27 male patients ranged in age from 21 to 63 years, with an average ('mean') age of 41 years. The 36 female patients ranged in age from 22 to 56 years, with an average age of 40 years. The age range for the normal volunteers was 19 to 48 years, with an average age of 32 years. The volunteers were personnel at the same hospital as that where the chronic fatigue syndrome patients were seen. Each blood sample was spun in a test tube at high speed (centrifugation) to separate out the heavier red blood cells (at the bottom of the tube) from the straw-coloured lighter plasma (at the top of the tube), with a thin layer of white blood cells in between. The red blood cells from each sample were then carefully taken out of the tube, washed in salt solution, and frozen. The frozen red blood cell samples from each patient were sent to Dr Mehar Manku and Nancy Morse-Fisher for expert chemical analyses of the fatty acid levels.

Dr Mehar Manku is someone I have known since the latter half of the 1990s, when we were both scheduled to give lectures on fatty acids at a meeting in Amman, Jordan. His professional career started off in Nairobi, Kenya, when he became a PhD student under David Horrobin, who had been appointed to the first professorship of physiology at the university there. After completing his doctorate, Dr Manku followed Professor Horrobin to Scotia Pharmaceuticals plc, and then to Laxdale Ltd (based in Stirling, Scotland). He is undoubtedly one of the world's leading experts on fatty acids and, in 2003, was appointed to the position of editor-in-chief of the prestigious international journal *Prostaglandins, Leukotrienes and Essential Fatty Acids*. I met Nancy Morse for the first time at the Brain Phospholipids Conference in 2003, when she travelled over from Canada, following the untimely and tragic death of Professor Horrobin on the first day of April 2003.

Dr Mehar Manku and Nancy Morse-Fisher analyzed fatty acid levels in the red blood cell samples without knowing which ones were from chronic fatigue syndrome patients and which from normal volunteers; the samples were coded and Mehar and Nancy were not privy to this code while carrying out the analyses.

Fatty acids are very important indeed to the proper functioning of our bodies. The whole of the next chapter is devoted to a description to them and their role in the treatment of chronic fatigue syndrome/M.E. If you are unfamiliar with any of the terminology used here ('omega-3 fats', 'omega-6 fats'), things will be clearer after you have read Chapter 4. Technical terms are also explained in the Glossary at the back of the book.

The results that Mehar and Nancy sent back to Professors Behan, Behan and Horrobin were striking once the sample codes were broken. Looking at all the omega-3 and omega-6 fatty acids that were investigated in the red blood cells, it turned out that the average levels were actually lower in the chronic fatigue syndrome group compared with the normal volunteer group. The values found are shown in Table 1. In some cases the chronic fatigue syndrome levels were so much lower that they were counted as being 'statistically significant'.

When scientists say that a finding is statistically significant, they mean that the result found was unlikely to have occurred by chance. Let us look at a rather contrived example. Normally if you toss an unbiased or fair coin in the air, then all things being equal there is a one in two chance that it will land with the head uppermost ('heads').

Table 1 Average levels of red blood cell fatty acids in 63 chronic fatigue syndrome patients and 32 normal volunteers (from Behan, Behan and Horrobin, 1990). (The values are given as milligrams per 100 milligrams of lipid.)

Fatty acid	Average value in 32 normal volunteers	Average value in 63 chronic fatigue syndrome patients
Omega-6 fatty acids		
Linoleic acid	15.2	14.0
GLA	1.7	1.6
AA	17.9	16.5
Adrenic acid	2.2	1.7
Total omega-6	37.8	33.5
Omega-3 fatty acids		
EPA	1.4	1.1
DPA	2.6	2.6
DHA	6.3	6.1
Total omega-3	10.4	10.0

There is also a corresponding one in two chance that it will land as 'tails'. (For purposes of simplicity, I am here ignoring the slight chance that the coin might land on its edge.) Now suppose you are given a biased coin that is weighted to make it come up 'heads'. You are asked to check whether or not this coin is biased. Suppose, further, that the only way you are allowed to carry out this test is by tossing the coin. Well, you toss the coin once, and the result is heads. This does not really prove anything at all, as there is a one in two chance that you would have got heads if the coin were unbiased. However, if you had decided to carry out a trial in which you tossed the coin three times, you would have got a result of three consecutive heads. A question you could now ask yourself is: 'How likely is it that I could get three or more consecutive heads purely by chance if the coin is unbiased?' Well, the chances of getting one head purely by chance with a fair coin are one in two, or one-half. So the chances of getting three heads purely by chance with a fair coin are (one-half) times (one-half) times (one-half). This is one-eighth. So there is a one in eight chance of getting a result of three consecutive heads (or a more extreme result – that is, more than three consecutive heads) purely by chance if the coin is unbiased.

Most scientists would consider that a chance of one in eight is well within the bounds of everyday possibility. The threshold that scientists set for considering that a result is unlikely to have occurred purely by chance tends to be around one in 20. (For those familiar with scientific papers, this is the origin of the famous 'P is less than 0.05' statement of statistical significance. The P stands for the probability (or chances) of the result occurring by chance. The 0.05 is the decimal representation of the fraction 1/20, which is the same as saying one in 20.)

Suppose now that you decided to carry out a much better trial to test whether or not the coin was fair by tossing it 10 times. This time, the biased coin lands heads uppermost on 10 consecutive occasions. The likelihood that this might happen by chance is:

(1/2) times (1/2) times (1/2) times (1/2) times (1/2) times (1/2) times (1/2) times (1/2) times (1/2) times (1/2).

This equals 1/1024. In other words, this result (or a more extreme result) had a less than one in a thousand likelihood of occurring by chance. Now you really would have reason to suspect that the coin might be biased.

Of course, the more times you tossed the coin, the more accurate your assessment; but in practice there is a limit to how far you can go. In a similar fashion, in scientific studies, there are practical factors that limit how far you can proceed. For example, Professor Behan's group would have obtained more accurate results if they had taken blood samples from every single person with chronic fatigue syndrome (postviral fatigue syndrome) in the whole world during a one-week period. This was clearly not practical. Similarly, when checking whether or not a coin is biased, you would obtain a higher accuracy if you were to spend your whole life tossing the coin every second of every day.

Let us now return to the blood results found by Professor Behan's group. In the following cases the chronic fatigue syndrome levels were so much lower that they were counted as being 'statistically significant'.

- AA (arachidonic acid) – this result (or a more extreme result) had a less than one in 20 likelihood of occurring by chance

- Adrenic acid – this result (or a more extreme result) had a less than one in 100 likelihood of occurring by chance

- The total omega-6 fatty acid level – this result (or one more extreme) had a less than one in 20 likelihood of occurring by chance.

Professor Malcolm Peet's group

A study that was superficially similar to the 1990 one of Professors Behan, Behan and Horrobin was published by Professor Malcolm Peet's group, based in Sheffield, England, in 1999 (Warren, McKendrick and Peet). Professor Behan's study used a clinical diagnosis (based on medical assessment rather than purely on strict, rigidly-defined research criteria) of postviral fatigue syndrome for patients to be included. In contrast, in Professor Peet's study the criteria used for including cases of chronic fatigue syndrome were the 'Oxford Criteria'. These differ from the revised CDC of Fukuda and colleagues that were described in Chapter 2. For example, the Oxford Criteria require fatigue to be the principal symptom and also include a subgroup of post-infectious fatigue syndrome in which the M.E.-like illness either specifically follows an infection or is associated with a current infection. The Oxford Criteria also specifically require patients to be suffering from fatigue 'which is severe, disabling and affects both physical and mental functioning'. In other words, whereas the revised CDC criteria of Fukuda and colleagues state that a major depressive illness would exclude a diagnosis of chronic fatigue syndrome, such a depressive illness would actually be part of chronic fatigue syndrome according to the Oxford Criteria.

In Malcolm Peet's study, the comparison of fatty acid levels in red blood cell membranes between 25 'chronic fatigue syndrome' patients and 25 normal control subjects (who were matched for age and gender) gave mostly different results to those in Peter Behan's 1990 study. This is not surprising, since the two studies used different diagnostic criteria. In particular, this time none of the comparisons between the patient group and the control group was strictly 'statistically significant'. The most significant result was the finding that the level of the important omega-3 fatty acid known as EPA (eicosapentaenoic acid; see Chapter 4) was lower in the patient group than in the control group. (Of the total phospholipids, on average EPA represented 0.55 in the patients, compared with 0.83 in the controls. This result (or one more extreme) was likely to occur by chance only six times in 100. Conventionally a rate of five times or less in 100 is counted as 'statistically significant'.)

Brain biochemistry

You might have wondered why the researchers who carried out the preceding two studies showed such an interest in the omega-3 and omega-6 fatty acids in the membranes of *red blood cells*. Sure, tiredness may result from anaemia, but these studies were not comparing anaemic patients and normal volunteers. Given that, besides fatigue itself, important symptoms of chronic fatigue syndrome can include problems with short-term memory and/or concentration, headaches, unrefreshing sleep, and prolonged malaise after exercise (at least according to the revised CDC criteria), then surely, you might argue, these researchers should have been investigating the brain rather than red blood cells garnered from peripheral veins in the arm. Well, you would be absolutely right. In fact, this is what the researchers were trying to do all along. Let me explain.

We will see in Chapter 4 that the levels of certain omega-3 and omega-6 fatty acids in the membranes of cells in the brain have profound effects on the activity of the brain. Here is an example. I was once called upon to give a private lecture to the directors of a couple of companies that are involved in the nutrition and fatty acid business. I noticed some of them making careful notes as I explained the benefits of taking a combination of virgin evening primrose oil with ultra-pure EPA (an extremely important omega-3 fatty acid) in the form of a preparation that is completely free of DHA (another omega-3 fatty acid). In spite of the fact that one of the companies markets its own omega-3 preparation (which, unfortunately, contains DHA), it turned out that within a week most of the directors started to take the DHA-free preparation. (At the time of writing, there is just one preparation available that contains virgin evening primrose oil, ultra-pure EPA, and zero DHA.) Within another four to six weeks I was receiving unsolicited comments such as 'I know EPA works, Basant. I've been taking VegEPA for four weeks now and my sleep has never been so good. And just look at J..... His concentration and his mood are so much better since he started taking it.'

In other words, altering the omega-3 and omega-6 fatty acid levels in the membranes of brain cells, by taking pure EPA and virgin evening primrose oil, can improve short-term memory, concentration, energy levels, and sleep. (In fact, I know from personal experience that the sleep you enjoy really is very refreshing. I too take this combination of oils.)

So why not study the levels of these fatty acids in the brain cells themselves? For Peter Behan and his colleagues to have achieved this in 1989-1990, they would have had to obtain brain biopsy material (that is, a tiny slice of brain tissue) from living humans, and then send the frozen, processed cell membrane material to Mehar Manku and Nancy Morse-Fisher for analysis. You see the problem: it is clearly recognized, at this time, that it is absolutely unethical to carry out such an invasive investigation. (I say 'at this time' because there have been circumstances, sadly, when such investigations would have been sanctioned by the state. Just think of Nazi Europe, for example.)

However, all was not lost for pioneers such as Peter Behan and his colleagues. In theory, the incorporation, or loss, of omega-3 and omega-6 fatty acids into the membranes of brain cells is reflected by a similar incorporation, or loss, into the membranes of all other living cells in the body. Now, red blood cells are readily accessible, needing only a small blood sample to be taken, using a sterile needle and syringe, from a vein in the arm, say, with little or no pain or discomfort and no lasting ill-effects. The omega-3 and omega-6 fatty acid levels in the membranes of the red blood cells, in turn, give indices of the levels of these fatty acids in the membranes of the brain cells.

Around about the year 2000, it occurred to me that I was in the fortunate position of having access to a machine and to a technology that can now allow us to investigate the chemistry of the membranes of brain cells directly, in the living human brain, in a way that is totally safe and non-invasive. The machine was a magnetic resonance imaging scanner, or MRI scanner. The technology was spectroscopy, or, strictly speaking, neurospectroscopy (also known as cerebral magnetic resonance spectroscopy or cerebral MRS).

Neurospectroscopy

Spectroscopy is a powerful technique that allows us to obtain a highly accurate chemical fingerprint from an object that is either emitting electromagnetic waves of its own accord (for example, stars send out light waves) or because it has been placed in a magnetic field and subjected to some radio (or other) waves (for example, in the strong magnetic field of an MRI scanner). Take the inert gas element helium, for example. Now, helium makes up almost one per cent of the air all around us. (It is also the second most abundant element in the known universe, after hydrogen.) Yet it was not in the air about us that helium was first discovered by humans. Amazingly, helium was first discovered in the Sun! Hence the name of the element (from the Greek *Helios*, the pagan Sun 'god'.) In the nineteenth century, Joseph Lockyer adapted his telescope to make it possible to use a spectroscope. In 1868, a spectrum, or chemical fingerprint, was obtained from sunlight. Part of this spectrum was readily attributable to the presence of hydrogen gas in the Sun. However, a bright yellow emission line was also seen in the spectrum, which could not be simulated in a laboratory in London with any known substance. Lockyer hypothesized that this chemical spectral signature was caused by the existence of a then unknown new element in the Sun, which he called helium. In the same year, Pierre Janssen of France also made the same spectroscopic discovery. In 1895, Sir William Ramsay isolated helium here on earth (from the mineral cleveite) and so confirmed that Lockyer's putative element really did exist. Lockyer was rewarded with a knighthood in 1897, becoming Sir Joseph Norman Lockyer.

To carry out spectroscopy examinations of the brain in living humans, we use an MRI scanner. This is usually a long, tunnel-like machine that operates at many tens of thousand times the strength of the earth's magnetic field. It is perfectly safe to be examined inside such a scanner, so long as you do not have any metallic objects on your person or inside your body. Examples of the former might be keys, paper clips and hair clips. The strong magnetic field could easily make such objects move at high speed, with the possibility of injury occurring. Examples of metallic objects inside the body include artificial heart pacemakers, cerebral aneurysm clips, metal implants, artificial implanted pumps and certain types of intrauterine contraceptive devices (IUCDs, also known as 'the coil'). These might move or fail to work properly as a result of entering the strong magnetic field environment of an MRI scanner. It is also important not to carry an object into the scanner area that contains information encoded on a magnetic medium such as a magnetic strip. A physicist at my place of work once had difficulty explaining how his credit card had come to be completely wiped of information from its magnetic strip after he had inadvertently kept it on his person when entering the high field zone.

So long as there are no metallic objects on or in a person, it is perfectly safe to be scanned in an MRI scanner. In particular, unlike X-ray machines, CT (computerized tomography) scanners or PET (positron emission tomography) scanners, with MRI scanners there is absolutely no exposure to ionizing radiation. The scanner can be a bit noisy, however. For that reason, subjects being scanned are asked to wear hearing protection, usually in the form of ear plugs and large headphones that cover each ear.

Usually when the brains of patients are scanned in most MRI scanners, the purpose is to obtain high-resolution pictures of the anatomy of the different parts of the brain. By programming the computer that is part of the MRI scanner in a special way, it is possible instead to obtain spectra. That is, it is possible to obtain detailed information about the chemistry of different parts of the living brain. In practice, if spectroscopy of the brain is to be carried out, then it makes sense also to obtain pictures of the anatomy of the brain first. That way, details can be sent to the scanner of the exact position in the brain from which chemical information is to be collected.

The first major neurospectroscopy studies were published around 1990. These were studies in conditions such as schizophrenia, multiple sclerosis and brain tumours. However, ten years later, I was not aware of any systematic neurospectroscopy studies comparing the chemistry of the brain in chronic fatigue syndrome with that in normal volunteers. So when I suggested such a study to some of my colleagues, with some of whom I had already been carrying out electrophysiological studies in chronic fatigue syndrome, they readily agreed.

The Hammersmith study

In 2002, my colleagues and I published the first systematic neurospectroscopy study of chronic fatigue syndrome, using one of the MRI scanners available to us at Hammersmith Hospital, London. A large team of professionals with various areas of expertise was involved in carrying out this investigation, as is evident from the list of the authors of this paper: Basant Puri (the author); Serena Counsell (a radiographer with expertise in MRI and neurospectroscopy); Dr Rashid Zaman (a psychiatrist who has been involved in several studies on chronic fatigue syndrome); Dr Janice Main (a senior lecturer and consultant physician with an expertise in infectious diseases and chronic fatigue syndrome); Alan Collins (an engineer with many years of experience with MRI scanning technology); Professor Joseph Hajnal (a physicist with a particular expertise in MRI); and Dr Nick Davey (a senior lecturer in neuroscience with a special interest in adaptation and reorganization of motor control in the brain and spinal cord). We recruited eight patients who met the revised CDC criteria of Fukuda and colleagues for chronic fatigue syndrome. They had an average (mean) age of a little under 43 years. We also recruited eight normal volunteers, who had an average age of just over 40 years. A particular form of neurospectroscopy, known as proton neurospectroscopy, was carried out in all 16 subjects. The brain has an outer layer of grey matter, known as the cortex, which surrounds the inner white matter. We obtained spectral information about the chemistry of the outer cerebral cortex.

The results of the study showed a clear difference in the chemistry of the brain between the chronic fatigue syndrome patients and the normal volunteers. In the back part of the brain is a region known as the occipital cortex. This is shown in the simple sketch of the brain that appears in Figure 1. Here, we found that the level of a particular chemical was much higher in the chronic fatigue syndrome patients than in the normal volunteers. This chemical was choline. We measured the ratio of choline to that of another chemical, creatine, which is known to remain relatively stable between subjects. Whereas the ratio of choline to creatine in the occipital cortex was 0.76 in the normal volunteers, it was much higher at 0.97 in the chronic fatigue syndrome patients. (This (or a more extreme) difference was 'statistically significant', as it would occur by chance only eight times in a thousand.)

This was the first time that a systematic study had been carried out into the chemistry of the living brain in patients with chronic fatigue syndrome and in matched normal volunteers. The study had

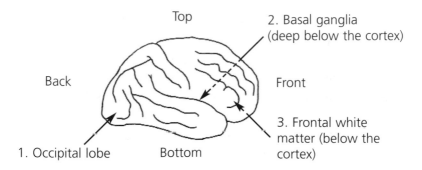

Figure 1. The location in the brain of (1) the occipital lobe (Hammersmith study), the basal ganglia (Chaudhuri study), and the frontal white matter (Tomoda study). The right side of the brain is shown.

given a clear-cut result. What did the result mean? There was one obvious explanation, namely, that there was a problem in respect of the turnover of omega-3 and omega-6 fatty acids in the membranes of the cells of that part of the brain that we had investigated.

There was a problem with this explanation, however. I was gaining a reputation for finding fatty acid changes in several brain diseases, including depression and Huntington's disease. So here I was, once again, with evidence suggesting the same in chronic fatigue syndrome. I felt I needed to be sure that my interpretation was not unduly biased by my knowledge of fatty acids. So I took the results and showed them in turn to two colleagues in our department, both of whom are experts in spectroscopy (each with a doctorate in this area), and neither of whom was involved in this study, without first telling them my own conclusions. The first expert was Dr Jimmy Bell. He had no hesitation in suggesting that our results related to an abnormality in fatty acid turnover in the patient group. Then I showed the results to Dr Jane Cox, who had actually taught me most of what I knew about spectroscopy a few years earlier. She not only also drew the same conclusion, but took me to her office where she found a copy of a scientific journal called *NMR in Biomedicine*, from 1992. She picked it up and turned to page 226. Here was an article by Ruiz-Cabello and Cohen in which they had described the meaning of a raised choline level: abnormal membrane phospholipid metabolism. In other words, a change in the turnover of fatty acids in the cell membranes. I was now satisfied with the conclusion, and we sent the paper off to the journal *Acta Psychiatrica Scandinavica*, in August 2001. This journal accepted the paper in March 2002 and duly published it in September 2002.

Other neurospectroscopy studies

In September 2002, soon after publication of our chronic fatigue syndrome neurospectroscopy paper, I received a telephone call from a senior lecturer in clinical neurosciences based at the University of Glasgow and Southern General Hospital, Glasgow, Scotland. He was Dr Abhijit Chaudhuri. He explained that he had read our Hammersmith Hospital/Imperial College paper, and that his group had a particular interest in our results. The reason was that they had also carried out a proton neurospectroscopy study in chronic fatigue syndrome. In fact, they had also scanned eight chronic fatigue syndrome patients and eight normal volunteers in their study, just as we had done. They had looked at another region of the brain, known as the basal ganglia, and, sure enough, they too had found a significant difference between the chronic fatigue syndrome patients and the normal volunteers: the choline level was increased in the chronic fatigue syndrome patients. So here we were, with two studies carried out using the same technology in two different centres and with the same numbers of chronic fatigue syndrome patients and normal volunteers, both of which showed an increase in choline in the brain. (In the next chapter we shall see how these findings can be caused by viral infections affecting the turnover of lipids in the brain.)

Dr Chaudhuri explained that he and his colleagues had presented their findings earlier that year at the main annual international conference in the MRI world, *The International Society for Magnetic Resonance in Medicine*. This had been the tenth annual scientific meeting and had been held between the 18th and 24th of May 2002 in Honolulu, Hawaii, in the United States of America. I apologized for my lack of familiarity with the work of Dr Chaudhuri's group; I had not attended the Honolulu meeting, having decided that the jet lag might not be good for my health, and in any case, I had submitted our paper the previous year, in August 2001.

Abhijit Chaudhuri went on to tell me something else that was also very interesting. Did I know that, although we at the Hammersmith had published the first systematic neurospectroscopy study of chronic fatigue syndrome comparing them with normal volunteers, there had been a series of three case studies using neurospectroscopy that had been previously published by a Japanese group? This was news to me, and I rapidly familiarized myself with the details of this paper. It was written by Akemi Tomoda and colleagues and published in the journal *Brain and Development* in the year 2000. They had scanned three children suffering from chronic fatigue syndrome, aged between 11 and 13 years, using proton neurospectroscopy. They had looked at the chemistry in the white matter at the front of the brain (the frontal white matter). For comparison, they had used data from 20 controls. One result stood out. Compared with an average value for the choline to creatine ratio of 1.09 in their controls in the frontal white matter, the corresponding values in the three children with chronic fatigue syndrome were as follows:

- Case 1 (an 11-year-old girl): 4.28

- Case 2 (a 12-year-old girl): 2.18

- Case 3 (a 13-year-old boy): 3.32.

As the authors themselves put it, 'The MR spectroscopy (MRS) study revealed remarkable elevation of the choline/creatine ratio in the patients with CFS.' So here too was a study (albeit not systematic) also showing an increased choline level in the brain (this time in the frontal white matter) in chronic fatigue syndrome.

In due course, Dr Chaudhuri's paper was published in the journal *Neuroreport* in February 2003. (The increase in choline that they found in the brain in chronic fatigue syndrome was highly 'statistically significant', with a result as big (or bigger) likely to occur by chance less than one in a thousand times.)

Gene expression

In 2005, my colleague Dr Jonathan Kerr and his group at Imperial College London published a study in the *Journal of Clinical Pathology* (Kaushik and colleagues, 2005). They studied white blood cells from 25 patients who had chronic fatigue syndrome diagnosed according to the CDC revised criteria and 25 normal blood donors who were matched for age, gender and geographical location.

Our genetic information is encoded in DNA in the form of genes on our chromosomes. Different genes contain the instructions to make different proteins. If more of one particular protein needs to be made, then the gene(s) for that protein is (are) 'expressed' more strongly. Interestingly, Kerr and colleagues found that, of the 9,522 genes they looked at, 15 showed increased expression, and one showed reduced expression in the CFS patients.

Their results suggested activation of T cells and changes in the function of nerve cells and mitochondria (the organelles in a cell that act as its powerhouses). Reporting on these findings in the 21st July issue of *New Scientist*, Rowan Hooper found that one of the gene products, EIF4G1, is involved in protein production in mitochondria. It is hijacked by some viruses, so cells may compensate by ramping up gene expression. This fits with the idea that CFS is sometimes triggered by viruses such as Epstein-Barr, Q fever, enteroviruses and parvovirus B19.

Not all in the mind

We have seen that, in spite of the 'psychosomatic' or 'hysteria' label, there is strong evidence that chronic fatigue syndrome is not a condition that is 'all in the mind'. The evidence, from a consideration of viral infections, changes in the immune system, blood fatty acid levels, and brain biochemistry, is compelling from each of these sources. We shall see, however, that all these results can be brought together into one overall model. This model is not only consistent with the findings described in this chapter, but it also provides a strong pointer to a suitable, natural treatment. Before we can discuss any of this, we need to familiarize ourselves with certain aspects of the subject of fatty acids.

4
How and why fatty acids can help

What are fatty acids?

Cell membranes

All our organs are made of tissues, which in turn are made of cells. Cells are the structural and functional units of all living organisms, including humans. There are many different types of cell in our organs. For example, in the brain there are neurones (brain cells) and glial cells. In the blood there are red blood cells and white blood cells.

All our living cells have a double-layered boundary called the cell membrane. These membranes also surround certain structures inside cells, called organelles. Examples of organelles include the mitochondria (which are the powerhouses of the cell) and the nucleus (which contains the genetic information of the cell in the form of DNA or deoxyribonucleic acid). The double-layered membrane around the nucleus is called the nuclear envelope.

Figure 2 is a diagram that shows the structure of a typical cell membrane.

Phospholipids

Cell membranes are made of two layers of molecules called phospholipids. A close-up of one of these phospholipid molecules is shown in Figure 3.

Each phospholipid molecule has a water-loving ('hydrophilic'

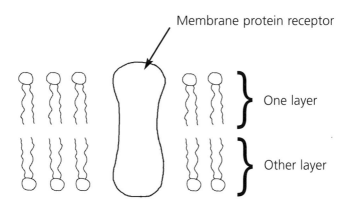

Figure 2. The structure of a typical cell membrane.

or 'polar') head component. A typical head component is choline, which we met in the previous chapter. Attached to the polar head component are two tails. These tails are water-hating ('hydrophobic'). Each tail is a fatty or lipid molecule called a fatty acid. As a result of the fact that the polar head components are attracted to water whereas the fatty acid tails are water-hating, the phospholipid molecules arrange themselves in the manner shown in Figure 2. That is, they form a double-layer, in which the polar head components face outwards, towards the watery environment of the fluid outside the cell and the watery environment of the fluid (cytoplasm) inside the cell. Meanwhile, the fatty acid tails are in a stable position by lying in a fatty environment away from the more watery environments just outside and inside the cell (or organelle).

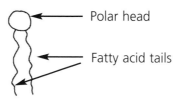

Figure 3. A close-up of a phospholipid molecule.

Fatty acids

Fatty acids are the water-hating fatty tails shown in Figures 2 and 3. In cell membranes, they tend to be long molecules, made up mainly of carbon and hydrogen atoms. Most of the bonds between adjacent carbon atoms in a fatty acid molecule are known as single-bonds. Occasionally, stronger double-bonds occur. For those of you with an interest in chemistry, Figure 4 shows the difference between a single-bond and a double-bond.

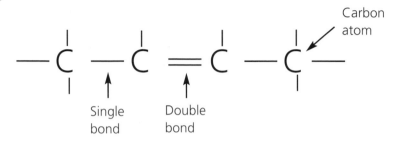

Figure 4. The difference between a single-bond and a double-bond between carbon atoms.

Fatty acids vary according to the total number of carbon atoms, the total number of double-bonds, and the positions of the double-bonds. Those fatty acids that have their first double-bond starting at the sixth carbon atom from a particular end of the molecule are known as omega-6 fatty acids. Similarly, those fatty acids that have their first double-bond starting at the third carbon atom from a particular end of the molecule are known as omega-3 fatty acids. These are very important molecules. Doubtless you will have come across the advice of the American Heart Association (published as *AHA Scientific Statement: Fish Consumption, Fish Oil, Omega-3 Fatty Acids and Cardiovascular Disease* in 1996) extolling the virtues of omega-3 fatty acids:

> Omega-3 fatty acids benefit the heart of healthy people, and those at high risk of — or who have — cardiovascular disease.

We recommend eating fish (particularly fatty fish) at least *two* times a week. Fish is a good source of protein and doesn't have the high saturated fat that fatty meat products do. Fatty fish like mackerel, lake trout, herring, sardines, albacore tuna and salmon are high in two kinds of omega-3 fatty acids, **eicosapentaenoic acid (EPA)** and **docosahexaenoic acid (DHA)**.

As well as preventing heart disease, omega-3 fatty acids have many other health benefits. These will be described in Chapter 7.

Meanwhile, it will help us understand better the role of fatty acids in chronic fatigue syndrome if we know a little about how the body obtains its supply of different omega-3 and omega-6 fatty acids.

How the body obtains omega-3 and omega-6 fatty acids

The diagram overleaf (Figure 5) summarizes the most important omega-3 and omega-6 fatty acids and how the body makes them. Basically, the first omega-6 fatty acid at the top of the left-hand chain, named linoleic acid, can be obtained from certain foodstuffs but cannot be made by our bodies. Once we have linoleic acid in our bodies (from food) in theory we have the chemical machinery to create all the succeeding omega-6 fatty acids below linoleic acid in the left-hand omega-6 chain. Thus, our cells can, in theory, convert linoleic acid into gamma-linolenic acid (GLA). In turn, GLA can be converted into dihomo-gamma-linolenic acid (DGLA). This in turn can be converted into arachidonic acid (AA), and so on.

Similarly, on the omega-3 side, the first omega-3 fatty acid at the top of the right-hand chain, named alpha-linolenic acid, can be obtained from certain foodstuffs but cannot be made by our bodies. Once we have alpha-linolenic acid in our bodies (from food) in theory we have the chemical machinery to create all the succeeding omega-3 fatty acids below alpha-linolenic acid that are shown in the right-hand omega-3 chain.

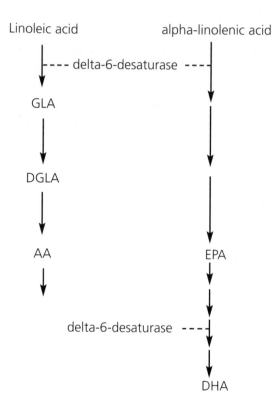

Figure 5. Omega-3 and omega-6 fatty acids.

Each succeeding step in the chain requires a particular naturally occurring enzyme. These enzymes catalyze chemical reactions that would otherwise take far too long to occur. As an example, consider what would happen if you were to eat a teaspoonful of ordinary white sugar (or sucrose, to give it its proper name). Assuming that you are not overweight and that you are exercising sufficiently to need some energy, then the sugar would react with oxygen (from the air you breathe in) and be converted into carbon dioxide gas and water, in your body, and in the process release a fair amount of energy, which you can use. However, if you do not consume the sugar and just leave it lying on your table, it is highly unlikely that it will undergo any such reaction, even though it is surrounded by air that is rich in oxygen. The same reaction that occurs rapidly in the body, because of the help of enzymes, is usually excruciatingly slow at room temperature without the presence of the enzymes. The enzyme required for the omega-3 and omega-6 fatty acid conversions are the same at any given stage in Figure 5. For instance, the enzyme that helps convert the omega-6 fatty acid linoleic acid into GLA is known as delta-6-desaturase. It is this same enzyme that aids the conversion of alpha-linolenic acid into the next omega-3 fatty acid in the chain.

Since linoleic acid and alpha-linolenic acid have to be provided by the diet and cannot be manufactured *de novo* by our bodies, they are known as essential fatty acids. The succeeding omega-3 and omega-6 fatty acids, particularly those with 20 or 22 carbon atoms, are known variously as long-chain polyunsaturated fatty acids, LC-PUFAs, highly unsaturated fatty acids, or HUFAs. These include dihomo-gamma-linolenic acid and arachidonic acid, on the omega-6 side, and eicosapentaenoic acid (EPA) and docosahexaenoic acid (DHA) on the omega-3 side.

What do omega-3 and omega-6 fatty acids do?

Structure of membranes

The omega-3 and omega-6 fatty acids have extremely important roles in maintaining the correct structure of cell membranes throughout the body. In particular, for a membrane to function properly, it needs to have sufficient levels of the omega-6 long-chain polyunsaturated fatty acid arachidonic acid, and the omega-3 long-chain polyunsaturated fatty acid docosahexaenoic acid. Without these fatty acids, cell membranes become more rigid, and this reduced flexibility is reflected in poorer or abnormal functioning of receptors that lie in the membranes. In turn, this means that communications between cells, including between brain cells, is impaired.

Eicosanoids

Even more importantly, two of the omega-6 long-chain polyunsaturated fatty acids, dihomo-gamma-linolenic acid (DGLA) and arachidonic acid (AA), and one of the omega-3 long-chain polyunsaturated fatty acids, namely eicosapentaenoic acid (EPA), act as the starting point for the manufacture, by the body, of many different vital substances, including:

- Families of prostaglandins

- Families of thromboxanes

- Families of hydroxy fatty acids

- Families of leukotrienes.

So important are these substances that whole textbooks have been written on individual members of each of these families. In essence, these substances, which collectively are called eicosanoids, are special types of hormones that act on nearby cells after being created, rather than being transported long distances in the body to cells and tissues that lie far away from their site of synthesis. They are involved in many processes that are important in maintaining the health and well-being of the body and in fighting disease, including:

- Blood clotting

- Regulating blood pressure

- Reproduction

- The response to disease or trauma (including inflammation responses, pain and fever)

- The secretion of acid by the stomach.

Sleep

When there is sufficient EPA (eicosapentaenoic acid) available to the body, it can be converted into natural sleep mediators. This is one of the reasons that my patients and acquaintances enjoy such wonderful, deep, refreshing sleep if they follow the advice to take a formulation each day that contains ultra-pure EPA (that is, EPA without any DHA). (In the next chapter, we shall consider the best ways to take fatty acids.)

Effect on viruses

The omega-3 fatty acid EPA (eicosapentaenoic acid) has a particularly important role in helping the body to combat viral infections. It turns out that EPA can actually kill viruses in the body, without harming us in the process. It does this in at least two ways.

First, EPA is itself directly viricidal. In other words, if you add small amounts of EPA solution to harmful viruses (such as the Epstein Barr Virus that causes glandular fever), then the EPA actually kills the virus.

Second, EPA is also indirectly viricidal. After being acted on by two sets of enzymes, known as COX (cyclo-oxygenase) and LOX (lipo-oxygenase), EPA is converted into families of interferons. These substances, in turn, have powerful antiviral actions.

Effects of viruses on omega-3 and omega-6 fatty acids

The last section might have left you slightly puzzled. How, you might be asking yourself, do viral infections ever manage to get a foothold in our bodies if they are susceptible to destruction by EPA? The answer is that in order to establish themselves in human bodies, viruses such as the Epstein-Barr virus need to stop our bodies from producing eicosanoids, and, in particular, EPA.

Suppose you were the general in command of a viral invasion force. Where are the weakest parts of the human line of defence that you should try to hit? If you turn back to Figure 5, you will readily see that if a viral species were to block the very first enzyme that our cells use to manufacture long-chain polyunsaturated fatty acids, then it would effectively block the production of all eicosanoids and would, in particular, block the synthesis of EPA. This would mean that the human body would not be able to use its EPA-based defences against the invading viruses

This is precisely what such viruses do. They stop that first enzyme (which you may remember is called delta-6-desaturase) from working properly, and so the poor cells and tissues of the human body are left essentially defenceless against the onslaught from the invading viruses, which are now free to reproduce rapidly and wreak havoc on the 'host'.

There are many other effects of this viral strategy that the human body has to endure as it loses the war against the invading viruses. Unable to make sufficient quantities of EPA, the human body is no longer able to manufacture sufficient quantities of the EPA-based natural sleep mediators. As a result, the body does not get enough deep refreshing sleep and ends up tired and even less able to resist the viruses. The lack of DGLA, arachidonic acid and EPA also means that the body cannot produce enough eicosanoids, and so the general health and well-being of the body suffers. The body cannot mount proper immune response measures against the invader, and has to endure long bouts of painful sore throats, and enlarged and tender neck (cervical) and armpit (axillary) lymph glands. EPA and certain eicosanoids normally help to keep our joints working properly and 'well-oiled'; their disappearance means that the body has to endure pains (arthralgia) in many different joints.

If these consequences were not bad enough, there is even worse to come. Blocking that first enzyme (delta-6-desaturase) also means that cell membranes cannot get enough arachidonic acid and docosahexaenoic acid so that they become more rigid and lose their normal flexibility. The effects on the protein receptor molecules that lie in the cell membranes are profound; the size and shape of these receptors change so that they no longer accept and pass on signals in the right way. Communication between cells is impaired. It would be like an enemy hitting our satellite and radar communications during a war. The results of this in the human brain are cognitive defects, such as problems with short-term memory and with concentration.

These results will sound familiar to any reader who is suffering from chronic fatigue syndrome. They constitute key symptoms and signs of this disease.

From the point of view of neurospectroscopy, there is yet another action of viruses that is particularly interesting. Carrasco published a chapter entitled *Modification of membrane permeability by animal viruses* in the 1995 book *Advances in Virus Research, Volume 45* in which the observation was made that certain molecules in the membrane of viruses induce particular changes in the permeability of the infected (human) cell membranes. In turn, this causes special enzymes (called phospholipases) to be activated. The result is that the phospholipids in the human cell membranes break down and release the water-loving head groups mentioned in the last chapter, including choline. In other words, a major viral infection would be associated with an increased level of choline on spectroscopy. As we saw in the previous chapter, this is exactly what has been found in the brain in chronic fatigue syndrome.

Viral model

The above description of the expected effects of a viral infection are consistent with a model in which a long-term viral infection is considered to be the primary cause of chronic fatigue syndrome.

Such a viral model also fits in perfectly with the evidence we looked at in the previous chapter of chronic fatigue syndrome not being 'all in the mind'. As a reminder, this evidence was fourfold:

- Viral infections

- Changes in the immune system

- Blood fatty acid levels

- Brain biochemistry.

The first of these, the evidence consistent with viral infections, is clearly consistent with a viral model of chronic fatigue syndrome.

The second consisted of well-documented changes in the immune system (reduced natural killer (NK) cell activity, reduced Th1 cell activity, increased Th2 cell activity and increased Tc cell activity), which are also consistent with a pre-existing long-term viral infection, to which the immune system is reacting.

The third type of evidence was from blood fatty acid levels. The large study by Professors Behan, Behan and Horrobin found that chronic fatigue syndrome was associated with reduced levels of arachidonic acid, adrenic acid (which is an omega-6 derivative of arachidonic acid) and total omega-6 fatty acids. In the later study by Professor Peet's group, the patient group (defined by the Oxford criteria) had a lower level of EPA. In neither study was there any reduction in the omega-3 and omega-6 essential (precursor) fatty acids linoleic acid and alpha-linolenic acid. As indicated earlier in this chapter, these results are consistent with a viral infection that blocks the first enzyme, delta-6-desaturase.

The fourth type of evidence was in the form of direct measures of brain biochemistry in chronic fatigue syndrome using neurospectroscopy. The key finding from two systematic studies and one set of case studies was an increased level of choline in the brain in this disease. As mentioned above, this is precisely what we would expect to see following a major viral infection.

How to defeat the viruses

We have seen that several lines of evidence point to a viral model of chronic fatigue syndrome. We have also seen how viruses can cause the symptoms of chronic fatigue syndrome, by their inhibition of the enzyme delta-6-desaturase. What we now need to do in the war against the viruses is to find a way to outflank their attack on our vulnerability at the delta-6-desaturase enzyme step.

Let us look carefully at Figure 5 (see page 50) again, which shows the position of the delta-6-desaturase step. By blocking delta-6-

desaturase, the viruses are stopping the invaded human bodies from making DGLA, arachidonic acid and EPA. So a way of outmanoeuvring the viruses would be to bypass the delta-6-desaturase step altogether, and prime the invaded human body with large amounts of DGLA, arachidonic acid and EPA. On the omega-6 side, we could simply give GLA, as this is easy to obtain (from evening primrose oil and starflower oil, for example). The GLA can then be readily converted into DGLA (via the enzyme elongase), and the DGLA can be readily converted into arachidonic acid (via the enzyme delta-5-desaturase). (The enzymes elongase and delta-5-desaturase are not usually inhibited by the viruses that inhibit delta-6-desaturase.) On the omega-3 side, we need EPA, and we can simply take pure EPA.

So an ideal combination is to give either evening primrose oil or starflower oil with EPA. We shall see in the next chapter that the best combination is virgin (cold-pressed, non-raffinated) evening primrose oil together with ultra-pure EPA (in a formulation that is completely free of the omega-3 fatty acid DHA).

Meanwhile, this is now a good point at which to look at the results of studies investigating the treatment of chronic fatigue syndrome with omega-3 and omega-6 fatty acids.

Studies of omega-3 and omega-6 fatty acids in the treatment of chronic fatigue syndrome

To date, there have been three major studies that have looked at the treatment of chronic fatigue syndrome with omega-3 and omega-6 fatty acids. The first was by Professors Behan, Behan and Horrobin in Glasgow, Scotland. The second was by Professor Malcolm Peet's group in Sheffield, England. The third set of studies has been carried out by me at the Hammersmith Hospital in London.

The Glasgow study

Mention has already been made, in Chapter 3, of the study of blood levels of omega-3 and omega-6 fatty acids in chronic fatigue syndrome and normal volunteers by Professor Peter Behan, Professor Wilhelmina Behan and Professor David Horrobin. This study of blood fatty acid was part of a systematic trial of the effects of treatment with omega-3 and omega-6 fatty acids in chronic fatigue syndrome, or post-viral fatigue syndrome as it was called at the time. The study was published in 1990.

Altogether 63 patients, diagnosed as having postviral fatigue syndrome, were entered into this study. Of the 63, 27 were men (average (mean) age 41 years) and 36 were women (average age 40 years). Their symptoms fulfilled the following criteria:

- Present for at least one year

- Present for less than three years

- Overwhelming fatigue

- Fatigue made worse by exercise

- Muscle pain (myalgia)

- Depression

- Poor concentration

- Poor short-term memory.

In all cases, the precipitating factor was an illness that was associated with a fever, and with nasal, throat or gut symptoms, and that was severe enough to mean that all the patients had been confined to bed for several days at that time. All the patients had also suffered from palpitations, shooting pains in the chest and unsteadiness.

Prior to the illness, all the patients had considered themselves to have been in good physical health.

A thorough physical examination was carried out to help exclude any other illness that might account for the symptoms. Medical investigations that were performed included urine tests, blood tests (including electrolytes, a full blood count, liver function tests, muscle enzymes, and thyroid function tests), a chest X-ray, a tracing of the electrical activity of the heart (electrocardiography or an ECG), tests for evidence of infection by viruses, and electrical and biopsy studies of muscles.

The clinical trial of treatment with omega-3 and omega-6 fatty acids was designed to last for three months, with evaluations timed to take place at the beginning (the baseline measurements), after one month, and at the end after three months. Purely at random (actually in accordance with the results of tossing a coin), the 63 patients were assigned either to an 'active' treatment group (destined to receive capsules containing the mix of omega-3 and omega-6 fatty acids) or a 'placebo' group (destined to receive a placebo, that is, a set of capsules of identical appearance that did not contain omega-3 and omega-6 fatty acids or indeed anything thought to be potentially therapeutic). After this randomization procedure, it turned out that 39 patients had been allocated to the active group and 24 to the placebo group; these two groups were matched in terms of the average age of the patients and their ratio of males to females. Neither the patients nor the clinicians assessing them were aware of the group allocation until the end of the study; in other words, the study was 'double-blind'.

The symptoms measured at the beginning (the baseline measurements), after one month, and at the end after three months, were:

- Fatigue

- Muscle pain (myalgia)

- Dizziness

- Poor concentration

- Depression.

Each of these symptoms was measured on a scale from zero to three, as follows:

0. Absent

1. Mild

2. Moderate

3. Severe.

The scores (from zero to three) for each of the five symptoms were then added up, to give an overall index of the severity of the postviral fatigue syndrome on each of the three assessment occasions. On the second and third assessment times, each patient's overall condition was evaluated, to see whether, compared to their condition at the start of the study, they were:

- Worse

- Unchanged

- Better.

The active treatment used was eight capsules daily of the product Efamol Marine. Each capsule contained:

- 36 milligrams (mg) GLA

- 17 mg EPA

- 11 mg DHA

- 255 mg linoleic acid.

Each placebo ('dummy') capsule contained:

- 50 mg linoleic acid in liquid paraffin

- No other omega-3 or omega-6 fatty acids.

The capsules of the active treatment and of the placebo looked identical and were made of soft gelatine. All the capsules also contained a small amount of vitamin E to act as an antioxidant (otherwise fatty acids can deteriorate and start to smell rancid). The GLA in the active treatment capsules was derived from another product, called Epogam, which consisted of evening primrose oil, that is, oil from seeds of the species *Oenothera*. The EPA and DHA in the active treatment were derived from concentrated fish oil. In order to avoid patients being able to taste the difference between fish oil and liquid paraffin, and so possibly break the 'blinding' code before the end of the study, they were asked to swallow their capsules whole and not to chew them. They were also asked to take their eight capsules as two capsules four times per day.

Blood samples were taken from all the patients, and from 32 normal volunteers (who were personnel at the same hospital), in order to measure levels of omega-3 and omega-6 fatty acids in the red blood cells. These measurements, at the start of the study, have already been described in the last chapter. Blood samples for the same measurements were also taken from the patients at the end of the study (that is, after three months).

The results of the study were striking. This applied to the overall assessments made by the doctors (who were blind to whether the patients were taking the active treatment or the placebo) in consultation with the patients, and to the assessments of the five individual symptoms.

Let us look at the results after just one month. First we shall consider the results in the group which had been taking the active treatment of omega-3 and omega-6 fatty acids. They had the following changes in respect of their overall assessments compared with how they were at the start of the trial:

- Worse: none

- Unchanged: 26%

- Better: 74%.

Now we turn to the group of patients who had been taking the placebo. They had the following changes in respect of their overall assessments compared with how they were at the start of the trial:

- Worse: none

- Unchanged: 77%

- Better: 23%.

So, after just one month, almost three-quarters of the group treated with omega-3 and omega-6 fatty acids were better compared with just under a quarter of the placebo group. The difference between the results for the two groups was 'highly statistically significant'. The chances of seeing a difference as great as (or greater than) that found, by pure luck, was less than two in ten thousand.

Also at one month, the degree of improvement in each of the five symptoms assessed (fatigue, muscle pain (myalgia), dizziness, poor concentration, and depression) was greater for the group being treated with omega-3 and omega-6 fatty acids than for the placebo group. The improvement in muscle pain (myalgia) and the overall total score were great enough for both to count as being 'highly statistically significant'. At the end of the study, after three months, the improvements were even more striking. The group of patients with postviral fatigue syndrome who had been taking the active treatment of omega-3 and omega-6 fatty acids now had the following changes in respect to their overall assessments compared with how they were at the start of the trial:

- Worse: none

- Unchanged: 15%

- Better: 85%.

At the same time, after three months, the group of patients with postviral fatigue syndrome who had been taking the placebo capsules had the following changes in respect to their overall assessments compared with how they were at the start of the trial:

- Worse: 9%

- Unchanged: 75%

- Better: 17%.

So, after three months, 85% of the group treated with omega-3 and omega-6 fatty acids were better compared with only 17% of the placebo group. The difference between the results for the two groups was again 'highly statistically significant'. The chances of seeing a difference as great as (or greater than) that found, by pure luck, was less than one in ten thousand.

Also at three months, the degree of improvement in each of the five symptoms assessed (fatigue, muscle pain (myalgia), dizziness, poor concentration, and depression) was greater for the group being treated with omega-3 and omega-6 fatty acids than for the placebo group. The improvements in all five symptoms were great enough for all five to count as being either 'statistically significant' (in the case of poor concentration) or 'highly statistically significant' (in the cases of fatigue, muscle pain, dizziness, and depression). In contrast, in the group of patients that had received the placebo for three months, each of these five symptoms had worsened compared with the scores two months earlier.

The red blood cell membrane fatty acid levels showed a much greater shift towards normal in the group of postviral fatigue syndrome patients treated with the omega-3 and omega-6 fatty acids than in the group who had received the placebo capsules.

Professors Behan, Behan and Horrobin ended their landmark 1990 paper as follow:

> In conclusion, our study shows that a treatment for PFS [post-viral fatigue syndrome] based on a biochemical abnormality known to be produced by certain viral infections can lead to significant clinical improvement.

The Sheffield study

The red blood cell membrane fatty acid results from the more recent Sheffield study, published in 1999 by Drs Warren and McKendrick and Professor Peet, have been mentioned in the previous chapter of this book. This study was an attempt to replicate the 1990 Glasgow study we have just looked at, and formed the basis for the doctorate (PhD) of one of Professor Malcolm Peet's students. There were two fundamental differences between these two studies. One, mentioned in the last chapter, was that in the Sheffield study the Oxford Criteria were used to define chronic fatigue syndrome. Second, rather than liquid paraffin (in combination with linoleic acid), the placebo used by the Sheffield group was sunflower oil.

Fifty patients were entered into this study. They were selected from 98 consecutive referrals to the regional infectious diseases unit, and consisted of 21 men and 29 women aged between 18 and 59 years, with an average (mean) age of 37 years. All 50 patients were given a full physical and psychiatric examination, and blood screen.

Twenty-five normal volunteers, who were matched in terms of age and gender with the first 25 patients, were recruited from the staff and students based in the hospitals that were involved in this study. The results of comparing the red blood cell membrane fatty acid levels in these normal volunteers with those of the chronic fatigue syndrome patients have been described in Chapter 3.

As in the Glasgow study, patients were asked to score each of the same five symptoms (fatigue, muscle pain (myalgia), dizziness, poor concentration and depression) from zero to three as follows:

0. Absent

1. Mild

2. Moderate

3. Severe.

This assessment was carried out at the start of the study and then every month until the end of the study at three months. Again, the scores (from zero to three) for each of the five symptoms were added up, to give an overall index of the severity of the chronic fatigue syndrome on each of the four assessment occasions. At the time of each of these four assessments, a depression inventory was also filled in and patients were also asked about any side-effects of the treatment.

The treatment was the same as in the Glasgow study, taken as before as two capsules of Efamol Marine four times per day. This time, however, the placebo consisted of eight capsules daily of sunflower oil. Each sunflower oil capsule contained:

- 335 milligrams (mg) linoleic acid

- 2 mg alpha-linolenic acid

- 230 mg mono-unsaturated fatty acids.

There was no EPA or DHA in the placebo capsules. Both the placebo capsules and the Efamol Marine capsules were encased in gelatine and contained some vitamin E as an antioxidant.

The results of the study varied considerably from those of the Glasgow study. Leaving aside the red blood cell membrane fatty acid levels at the start of the study, which have been discussed in the last chapter, the main results were summarized by the authors as follows:

2) Symptomatology in both groups [that is, active and placebo] improved with time but there was no specific benefit from Efamol Marine. In fact patients on sunflower oil showed a trend towards greater improvement.

3) There were slight changes in the fatty acid composition of RBC [red blood cell] membranes after treatment but the differences between the treatment and placebo groups were generally not [statistically] significant.

Overall, then, this was a negative study that failed to demonstrate any benefit in chronic fatigue syndrome from Efamol Marine. The difference with the Glasgow study might be accounted for by the fact that different selection criteria were used. Also, it is possible that the sunflower oil might have had some therapeutic effects of its own, which would have negated the difference in response between the two groups. In addition, Efamol Marine is not the ideal combination of oils. I will say more about this in the next chapter.

The Hammersmith Hospital studies – detailed case report and MRI study

In this section I shall describe first a case of chronic fatigue syndrome that was investigated in great detail before and after treatment with fatty acids. Specialized testing using MRI scanning is described here. In the next section, I shall relate the clinical findings from a series of chronic fatigue syndrome patients who were treated with fatty acids.

The first study was a detailed case report involving MRI scanning. It was published in 2004 by Dr Basant Puri (the author), Miss Joanne Holmes (who was a research radiographer based at Hammersmith Hospital at the time of the study) and Dr Gavin Hamilton (a physicist with a particular expertise in matters relating to magnetic resonance).

A 25-year-old woman, whom I shall refer to as Elizabeth, who had suffered from medically confirmed chronic fatigue syndrome, was referred to me in early 2003. She had contracted a viral infection at the age of 19 years, and following this she was diagnosed as suffering from chronic fatigue syndrome. I saw Elizabeth for the first time, together with her parents, in March 2003. At that time she was suffering from chronic fatigue, intense lassitude, poor sleep (marked by great difficulty in getting off to sleep each night), low mood and muscle pain. She was almost totally confined to a wheelchair during her waking hours, needing assistance to reach destinations inaccessible to the wheelchair. The wheelchair itself had to be pushed by others; Elizabeth lacked the energy to move the wheelchair by herself. In fact, one of her parents had to push her wheelchair into my clinic.

I formally assessed the degree of her depression using a special rating scale called the Montgomery and Åsberg Depression Rating Scale. Then she was scanned in one of our MRI scanners to give me a very accurate assessment of the structure or anatomy of her brain.

From the point of view of the treatment of chronic fatigue syndrome, one of the problems with Efamol Marine was that it did not provide enough EPA, in my opinion. I therefore prescribed Elizabeth a course of omega-3 and omega-6 fatty acids that contained a far higher EPA dose than that delivered in the Glasgow and Sheffield studies described above. The supplement I chose was 'eye q' at a total dose of 10 capsules daily, taken as five capsules twice per day; at this stage the product VegEPA, the product I now use in clinical trials because it delivers an even higher EPA dose (without any DHA) was not available. Ten capsules of the supplement chosen in 2003 provided the following daily fatty acid doses:

- 100 milligrams (mg) GLA

- 930 mg EPA

- 290 mg DHA.

In addition, the preparation also supplied 16 milligrams of vitamin E daily.

When I saw Elizabeth again after 16 weeks, she was a transformed person. She and her mother both reported that her chronic fatigue began to go into remission, for the first time in over six years, between six and eight weeks after she started to take the omega-3 and omega-6 fatty acid supplementation. By 16 weeks, Elizabeth reported being more motivated, having a brighter mood and sleeping much better. Sixteen weeks earlier we had had to push her, in her wheelchair, to the changing area. This time, when I told her it was time for her to get ready for her follow-up MRI scan, to the amazement of those of my colleagues who had seen her the first time, Elizabeth simply got up from her wheelchair and walked totally unaided over 20 yards to the changing area and thence to the MRI scanner area. Some of my colleagues gave me a curious look; it was almost as if I had successfully told my patient to take up her bed and walk. For her own part, Elizabeth confirmed that she had indeed noticed that she was able to walk better. She reported that her depressed mood had lifted after taking the omega-3 and omega-6 fatty acid supplementation, and this was confirmed by the change in the ratings. When I had first seen her, in March 2003, Elizabeth's score on the Montgomery and Åsberg Depression Rating Scale was 27, which is high and consistent with a moderate to severe degree of depressed mood. After supplementation for 16 weeks, the score on this rating scale had fallen to a mere three, which was consistent with having almost no depressive symptoms or signs. Not everything had improved on this particular supplement, however: Elizabeth had not noticed any change in her muscle pain.

We re-scanned her brain in the same MRI scanner. I then used a special technique, which I had helped co-develop as part of my PhD doctorate thesis some years before, to assess in a very accurate way what had happened to the lateral ventricles of Elizabeth's brain. The ventricles are four 'spaces' within the core of the brain. The two largest ones are the lateral ventricles, with one projecting into each half (or hemisphere) of the brain. They are perfectly normal structures to have in the brain. They help make the cerebrospinal fluid (or CSF) which bathes and nourishes the brain from both within (inside the ventricles) and without. It is this cerebrospinal fluid that doctors take a sample of when they carry out a lumbar puncture or 'spinal tap' investigation. If someone is developing a dementing illness such as Huntington's chorea (or Huntington's disease) or Alzheimer's disease, the size of the lateral ventricles can become quite large, as the volume of actual brain tissue diminishes.

Normally, when someone's brain is scanned on two different occasions, as was the case with Elizabeth, it is virtually impossible to ensure that, in practice, the brain is in exactly the same position (to the nearest one hundredth of a millimetre in each spatial dimension) at both times. This means that, on looking at the MRI scans from the two occasions, for example in order to assess how the ventricles have changed in size, if at all, one is not comparing like with like. On the contrary, just slight shifts or slight rotations of the head on the second occasion, compared with the time of the first scan, can translate into rather large shifts and changes between the two sets of scans. Of course, this makes it difficult to tell from the final images whether or not small changes have occurred in the structure of the brain. This problem was successfully tackled at Hammersmith Hospital in the mid-1990s by Joseph Hajnal (now Professor of Physics at Imperial College London) and Graeme Bydder (at that time Professor of Radiology at Hammersmith Hospital and the Royal Postgraduate Medical School, and currently Professor of Radiology at the University of California at San Diego – UCSD).

Using the Hajnal/Bydder methodology as our foundation, during the second half of the 1990s I worked with an exceptionally talented computer expert, named Dr Nadeem Saeed, on a further development of the technique that would allow us to find a way of accurately measuring the amount of change that occurred in parts of the brain such as the lateral ventricles between successive MRI brain scans. We succeeded in creating this technique; I was awarded a PhD from Imperial College London for my efforts, while Dr Saeed left our department and went to work for a major British pharmaceutical company. (Interested readers can read a review of this technique published in the journal *Prostaglandins, Leukotrienes and Essential Fatty Acids* by Puri in 2004 – see the References at the end of this book.)

I applied this state-of-the-art technology to the scans of Elizabeth's brain taken before and then after 16 weeks' of supplementation with omega-3 and omega-6 fatty acids. The results were astonishing. At the time of the first scan, just before starting the supplementation, the volume of the lateral ventricles in her brain was 28 900 cubic millimetres (actually, 28 938 cubic millimetres was the exact figure the computer workstation program gave me). Now, normally, in a 25-year-old woman, I would not expect to see any change in the size of the brain, including the size of its lateral ventricles, over a period of just 16 weeks. Yet, from the MRI brain scan taken after 16 weeks' of supplementation, the highly accurate technique I had at my disposal gave me a figure for the volume of her lateral ventricles of 23 700 cubic millimetres (23 662 cubic millimetres being the exact figure the computer workstation program gave me this time). This represented an amazing 18% decrease in the volume of the lateral ventricles in just 16 weeks. By carefully studying contiguous 'slices' of Elizabeth's brain on a computer workstation, I could see that during those 16 weeks her brain tissue had actually increased in size. In other words, it seemed that the main reason that Elizabeth's lateral ventricles had decreased in size by 18% was to make room for the increase in the size of her brain tissue. This brain growth puts me in mind of a more recent chronic fatigue syndrome patient of mine who, in 2004, told me that before she had ever learnt of this report by me, she had told her doctor that, as a result of taking VegEPA capsules daily, she felt sure she was experiencing brain re-growth.

Commenting on all these results, we included the following conclusions in our 2004 paper (published in the *International Journal of Clinical Practice*):

> Supplementation with a high-EPA containing essential fatty acid preparation was associated with the first remission for the patient of symptoms and signs of chronic fatigue syndrome in over six years. The patient has chosen to continue with this supplementation and, to date, no adverse side-effects have been observed.

> The relatively large reduction in lateral ventricular size is likely to be causally linked to the essential fatty acid supplementation, since phospholipids are important in the formation and remodelling of dendrites and synapses.

The Hammersmith Hospital studies – case series

In the first series of case reports from the Hammersmith, I reported on a series of four patients in the medical journal *Prostaglandins, Leukotrienes and Essential Fatty Acids* (Puri, 2004). The patients ranged in age from 20 to 56 years and were suffering from intractable chronic fatigue syndrome at the time they started taking the eye q supplement in 2002 to 2003 in doses ranging from 10 to 18 capsules daily, with an average of 12 capsules per day. All four patients showed improvement in their symptomatology, which started within 12 weeks of commencing the omega-3 and omega-6 fatty acid supplementation. The first patient commented as follows: 'The first thing is that the fogginess of the brain has gone completely'. The second commented that something was felt to be 'changing for the better in the lower part to the right side at the back of the brain', and that, 'for the first time a feeling of well-being [was experienced]'. The third patient commented that her 'relapses [had become] more spaced out', dropping from between four and 12 per month in the winter months before taking fatty acid supplementation to between one and three per month during the three winter months when supplementation was first taken. The fourth patient remarked that his relapses were 'not so severe; [I am] able to maintain normal awareness – this was [previously] a problem but has improved. Also [I am able to] communicate whilst in a relapse, this was not possible before treatment'.

In 2004, the best omega-3 and omega-6 fatty acid supplement ever to come to the market became available to patients with chronic fatigue syndrome. The reasons why this supplement is the best will be explained in the next chapter. I have looked at the records of the first 20 patients with previously intractable chronic fatigue syndrome who were put on this supplement. They were started on between four and eight VegEPA capsules daily. Of the 20, 17 experienced a remarkable level of improvement within three months. When I looked at the dose of the supplement they had taken, an interesting finding emerged. The first four patients had taken just four capsules daily. Of these four patients, one had improved within three months. The next 16 patients had taken either seven or eight capsules daily. All 16 of these patients had improved within three months. (These results have not yet been written up for publication in a medical journal at the time this book is being written.)

As a result of my clinical experience, I now recommend that patients start on eight capsules of the supplement each day. Eight VegEPA capsules taken daily deliver:

- 2 240 milligrams (mg) EPA

- 800 mg virgin evening primrose oil

- Zero DHA.

This represents the highest dose of EPA I have ever given to chronic fatigue syndrome patients. We shall see in the next chapter why the inclusion of virgin evening primrose oil and having a preparation that is DHA-free makes this an excellent formulation. The quotation in Chapter 1 is just one of the 16 cases.

The mother of a 23-year-old chronic fatigue syndrome sufferer wrote the following unsolicited letter to the manufacturer of the supplement just four weeks after her daughter had started taking it:

Dear Sir or Madam

Please find enclosed cheque and order for your product. I recently bought one month's supply of VegEPA for my daughter who suffers with M.E. I have to say that since taking VegEPA, my daughter Amanda who is 23 yrs old has had her first full nights sleep in three years. My husband and myself and family are delighted at this, as Amanda has been very poorly over the past three years. Amanda finds VegEPA very easy to digest and feels better than she did. I am very thankful that Dr Puri...

This letter has been reproduced with the permission of Amanda and her mother. After just another fortnight the improvement in symptoms had become even greater. Moreover, a long-standing rash across the chest, which had never previously responded to medical intervention, just disappeared. We shall see in Chapter 7 that improvements in the well-being of the skin are to be expected with a formulation such as the one taken by this patient. In September 2004, Amanda, her mother and I agreed to be interviewed by BBC Radio 4. This interview was broadcast on the programme *You and Yours*, as part of a special item on chronic fatigue syndrome.

Another typical example was the following e-mail sent to the manufacturer from a grateful client in Australia who had been suffering for years from chronic fatigue syndrome and had taken the supplement for approximately three months:

I am so much better than I have been – this time last year I was unable to walk to the bathroom unaided, could not sit up in bed to eat so had to do it lying down, and could only talk for about 5 minutes an hour. I couldn't read or watch tv, and when someone lent me some talking books, I listened for a few minutes and then my brain could no longer understand what was being said – sounded as if the narrator was speaking Russian. So to be feeling this much better is a miracle.

Enclosed with the VegEPA was a copy of your new brochure. I should like to send a few of these to my specialist who is going to try it on some of his other M.E./CFS patients.

5

How to take fatty acids

Having decided to take omega-3 and omega-6 fatty acids as a natural treatment for chronic fatigue syndrome, you are faced with a bewildering array of different omega-3 and/or omega-6 preparations, some of which contain concentrated fish oils (for the omega-3), and some of which contain evening primrose oil or starflower oil (for the omega-6). Then there are some so-called experts who claim that all you need to do is eat more oily fish. The aim of this chapter is to help you understand these issues better. With such understanding comes great clarity – by the end of the chapter you will find that you can see right through the forest of competing claims and counter-claims. You will have a clear understanding of the thought processes that have guided me into choosing a unique omega-3 and omega-6 fatty acid supplement that is delivering excellent results in clinical practice. You will also be able to evaluate any new products that may come on the market.

Evening primrose oil

What is it?

Evening primrose oil is extracted from seeds of the evening primrose plant (*Oenothera biennis*). This is a wildflower found growing naturally in Europe, North America, and parts of Asia. Its seeds have been used for centuries by American Indians. The common name evening primrose derives from the fact that the plant has pale yellow flowers which open in the evening.

Oil extracted from the seeds of the evening primrose plant are rich in the omega-6 long-chain polyunsaturated fatty acid GLA (gamma-linolenic acid). You will recall from the previous chapter that our cells should, in theory, be able to produce GLA from the dietary precursor linoleic acid, so long as the enzyme delta-6-desaturase is functioning properly.

The person who was probably most responsible for bringing evening primrose oil into popular use was the late Professor David Horrobin, who helped set up the company Efamol Ltd. and launched the evening primrose oil-based product Efamol. More on the history of evening primrose oil can be found in the excellent short book by Judy Graham, entitled *Evening Primrose Oil: Its Remarkable Properties and its Use in the Treatment of a Wide Range of Conditions*, first published in 1984.

Benefits

As we saw in the previous chapter, by by-passing any blocks to the functioning of the enzyme delta-6-desaturase, taking GLA allows our cells and tissues to produce adequate amounts of DGLA (dihomo-gamma-linolenic acid) and AA (arachidonic acid), which in turn are used to form various families of the important, health-promoting eicosanoids. Some of the benefits that have been attributed to taking GLA in the form of evening primrose oil include:

- Improvement of premenstrual syndrome (PMS, or premenstrual tension or PMT)

- Improvement of painful breasts (mastalgia)

- Improvement of certain skin conditions

- Improvement of the nails

- Improvement of the skin

- Improvement of nerve damage in diabetes mellitus.

Why virgin?

Rather than suggest that my patients go out and buy the cheapest evening primrose oil capsules they can find, I recommend that they take a special form of evening primrose oil, known as virgin evening primrose oil (as found in VegEPA capsules). Why?

Ordinary evening primrose oil preparations are made by processing the seed oil at relatively high temperatures and in other ways that remove some of the beneficial properties from the oil. In the same way that modern industrial processing of wheat grains strips away many nutritious and important substances (such as fibre, certain vitamins and minerals) to leave the pale, far less tasty, constipating 'food' we know as white flour, so modern industrial processing of evening primrose oil strips away much of the goodness and rich full flavour of the natural oil to leave what is, in essence, a pale imitation. To carry the analogy further, whereas most commercially available evening primrose oil preparations are like white flour, virgin (non-raffinated, cold-pressed) evening primrose oil is like wholemeal flour, complete with the nutrients still intact.

In 2004 I published a paper entitled *'The clinical advantages of cold-pressed non-raffinated evening primrose oil over refined preparations.'* For the purposes of this study, I started by looking at two common commercially available over-the-counter sets of capsules of evening primrose oil. On syringing out the contents of these capsules, I saw a pale, insipid-coloured (non-virgin, refined) evening primrose oil. However, I had a vial of a third evening primrose oil preparation available to me. This was of virgin evening primrose oil (exactly as contained in VegEPA capsules). Instead of the pale, straw-coloured liquid I was used to, the virgin evening primrose oil was a deep rich green colour, because it had not been refined. Analysis of this virgin evening primrose oil preparation replicated the results that had been published by a German group two years before. In 2002, Matthias Hamburger and his colleagues from the Institute of Pharmacy, Friedrich-Schiller-University Jena, in Jena and the Institute of Pharmacy, Humboldt-University Berlin, in Berlin, had published a paper in the *Journal of Agricultural and Food Chemistry* in which they had shown that virgin (cold-pressed, non-raffinated) evening primrose oil is rich in a group of compounds known as triterpines. In contrast, they had reported that commercial samples of (non-virgin) evening primrose oil only contained traces of triterpines.

Triterpines are naturally occurring compounds that help the body mop up dangerous 'free radicals', that enable our white blood cells to function better, and that help reduce the pain of arthritic joints. Since I believe that viral infections play an important part in causing chronic fatigue syndrome, it would make sense for patients with this disease to take virgin evening primrose oil rather than ordinary preparations.

Why not just eat more fish?

We have seen why I favour virgin evening primrose oil as the source of the omega-6 fatty acid GLA. When it comes to the omega-3 side of the equation, as we saw in the previous chapter, I strongly favour taking EPA. However, there is a school of thought that argues that we can obtain the EPA we need just by eating more fish. In principle, it is true that fish, particularly oily fish such as salmon, trout, herring, tuna, mackerel and sardines, are a good source of EPA. There are, though, at least two disadvantages to this approach.

First, in order to obtain a high enough quantity of EPA, you would have to eat a large amount of fish each day. I tend to start my chronic fatigue syndrome patients on a dose of omega-3 and omega-6 fatty acid supplementation that delivers over 2,000 milligrams of EPA daily. In order to obtain that from fish, you might have to consume around 400 grams of fresh tuna or trout each day, or perhaps around 200 grams of mackerel daily.

The second disadvantage is even more compelling. Humans have been busy polluting the rivers, seas and oceans of the world with toxins such as heavy metals (like lead, mercury and cadmium), dioxins (a generic term which covers polychlorinated dibenzo-p-dioxins and dibenzofurans) and PCBs (polychlorinated biphenyls). Heavy metals such as mercury and cadmium can be dangerous for the body, including the brain, while dioxins and PCBs have been linked to the possibility of causing illnesses such as cancer. Furthermore, although there may be a relatively low concentration of these pollutants in seawater, they tend to be concentrated by each successive level of the food chain. This means that, by the time top marine predators in the food chain such as trout and salmon are reached, the concentrations of these dangerous chemicals may have reached levels that are a million times greater than in the surrounding seawater

What about ordinary fish oil capsules?

Ordinary fish oil suffers from the same problem we have just mentioned: the risk from pollutants such as lead, mercury, cadmium, dioxins and PCBs. In fact, there are at least four reasons why the situation is even worse in respect of fish oil compared with just ordinary fish in the diet.

First, many of the harmful pollutants that are concentrated in the bodies of fish, such as dioxins and PCBs, are highly fat-soluble. This means that they are even more concentrated in fish oils (which, by definition, are oils and therefore fatty).

Second, we need to consider how fish oils tend to be extracted in industrial quantities from the bodies of fish. One method often used in industry is simply to squeeze the livers of the fish, and use (and sell) the liver oil thereby produced. A common example is cod liver oil, which has a good deal of EPA in it, and is extracted from the liver of cod. A major problem with this process is that in vertebrates such as fish (and, indeed, us), the liver is the main organ used for the detoxification of the blood. So, the liver oils can offer an even more concentrated concoction of dangerous pollutants. Another commonly used method is not to squeeze just the liver of the fish, but instead to squeeze the whole body of the fish, and collect the oil that comes out of the back passage. Needless to say, the alimentary tract (gut) is a very good source of the poisons of which the vertebrate body may wish to rid itself.

The third reason is that fish oil is rich in vitamin A. Adults who are healthy tend to have large stores of this vitamin in the liver. If taken in excess, vitamin A is toxic, and can even be fatal.

Unfortunately, in order to obtain the levels of EPA needed to treat chronic fatigue syndrome (between one and two grams of EPA daily), the amount of fish oil that has to be consumed could be dangerous. This is because the amount of vitamin A being consumed daily could easily reach the toxic range. Note that it is also possible to become vitamin A toxic from vegetables. There was a case in the 1990s of a man in Britain who drank huge amounts of carrot juice several times daily, every day. Eventually the toxic levels of vitamin A he was building up in his liver caused irreparable damage to this organ. He died from the high intake of vitamin A. (Note that the preparation VegEPA is completely free of vitamin A.)

The fourth reason is that, in addition to containing EPA, fish oil also contains DHA. In the next section you will see why you should avoid any supplements that contain DHA.

DHA

Why is a DHA-free supplement better?

With one exception, at the time of writing this book all the EPA-containing supplements available to the general public also contain the omega-3 long-chain polyunsaturated fatty acid DHA (docosa-hexaenoic acid). So why do some of the leading researchers in the field of lipids refuse to take supplements that contain DHA? There are several reasons.

The first reason we shall look at is a practical one. If a supplement contains both EPA and DHA, then it is likely that it is simply fish oil. The oil extracted from oily fish (whether from the liver or squeezed through the alimentary tract) tends to be rich in both EPA and DHA. But we have just seen why fish oil can be dangerous to our health, if it contains heavy metals and poisonous fat-soluble pollutants such as dioxins and PCBs. When a mass-produced fish oil preparation contains both EPA and DHA, it is far cheaper to make it by simply packing fish oil, than for manufacturers carefully to extract pure EPA and pure DHA and then put them together without any other components of the fish oil (including the pollutants). In contrast, in the case of the one product available to the general public that contains virgin evening primrose oil combined with EPA but no DHA whatsoever (namely, VegEPA), just ultra-pure EPA has been extracted from the fish oil, and everything else in the fish oil, including the DHA and the pollutants, has been discarded. It is rather like taking ordinary river water, and distilling off and collecting ultra-pure water from it. This water would be extremely safe to drink and would contain no pollutants. To follow through this analogy, the ultra-pure EPA would be to ordinary fish oil as ultra-pure water would be to ordinary river water.

A second reason why we should avoid supplements that contain DHA is that some of the leading researchers in the field have come to the conclusion that when ingested, the type of DHA that comes in supplements tends to inhibit many of the beneficial actions of EPA. (You may recall from the previous chapter how EPA is a direct precursor of many families of eicosanoids, and how it can also kill viruses and also form natural sleep mediators that promote deep, refreshing sleep.) The reason for this is not yet known. In fact, in general it has been found that as the ratio of EPA to DHA rises in the supplement used in clinical trials of certain conditions, such as depression and attention-deficit hyperactivity disorder (ADHD), the ability of the supplement to improve the condition also rises. At one extreme, using a completely DHA-free supplement will deliver excellent results. At the other extreme using pure DHA has never been found to work at all in depression or attention-deficit hyperactivity disorder. In fact, there have been double-blind trials of pure DHA in which the placebo has actually been found to be better than the DHA; in other words the DHA might even make patients worse.

As if these anti-DHA arguments were not enough, yet another reason is emerging for why we should avoid taking DHA in supplement form. In June 2004, Dr Thorlaksdottir, from the Department of Biochemistry and Molecular Biology, School of Medicine, University of Iceland, together with colleagues from other departments and from the Icelandic Cancer Society, presented some new results from a study that they had just completed but not yet published in a scientific or medical journal. They looked at the number of breaks in the DNA (deoxyribonucleic acid) molecules of the nuclei of certain white blood cells called peripheral blood mononuclear cells.

DNA makes up the genes and chromosomes of cells. It is important that DNA strands do not break, as this can mean that the programming of the cell might change ('mutate'). In turn, this means there might be a risk of cancer developing.

Dr Thorlaksdottir and her colleagues looked at these DNA breaks in 98 healthy women, whose average age was 46 years. A wide range of DNA damage was found in these subjects. Dr Thorlaksdottir and her colleagues also looked at red blood cell membrane levels of many different fatty acids, including omega-3 and omega-6 fatty acids, saturated fatty acids and monounsaturated fatty acids. In the case of just two of these fatty acids, there was a positive correlation between the level of the fatty acid and the amount of DNA damage. The two fatty acids were DHA and linoleic acid. The higher the red blood cell membrane level of either DHA or linoleic acid, the greater the level of DNA damage measured in the white blood cells. (There were no such statistically significant associations between DNA damage and dihomo-gamma-linolenic acid, arachidonic acid or EPA.)The conclusion that Dr Thorlaksdottir and her colleagues from the University of Iceland and the Icelandic Cancer Society came to was that:

These data suggest that dietary linoleic acid and DHA may be positively associated with DNA damage.

Dr Thorlaksdottir and her colleagues wondered if the mechanism of the DNA damage was the result of the way in which some fatty acids are prone to becoming oxidized, and that this oxidative damage might result in products (such as free radicals) that in turn could cause DNA damage. (Incidentally, this is another reason why the triterpines in virgin evening primrose oil – but not in ordinary processed evening primrose oil – are so helpful, as they can, as it were, mop up free radicals.)

Avoiding DHA from supplements is easy; you can just take the DHA-free supplement VegEPA. Fortunately, we do not have to worry too much about linoleic acid, as most of it is 'compartmentalized' soon after we absorb it.

Although Dr Thorlaksdottir and her colleagues had not

published their work formally in a journal by the time I wrote this book, they did manage to present their work in abstract form at a conference (see the References section at the end of this book). Worryingly, their abstract began with the following sentence:

> DNA modification is believed to be an important step in carcinogenesis [that is, in causing cancer].

But don't we need DHA?

Sometimes, when I explain to patients the virtues of taking a supplement that contains a combination of virgin evening primrose oil with ultra-pure EPA, that crucially is completely DHA-free, they worry about the fact that they have read articles stating that we need DHA. Will they not end up deficient in DHA, they wonder.

It is perfectly true that DHA is useful to the body – but only in a limited way. If you re-read part of Chapter 4, you will recall that the main function of DHA in the body is a structural one. It helps form the correct, flexible, structure of membranes that both bound cells and bound organelles inside cells. If you take ultra-pure EPA (without any DHA), then your body can readily make DHA as and when it is needed, in just the right places where it is required, from the EPA you have taken. Just glance again at the diagram on page 50 (Figure 5) to see how the body can do this. (Recall that EPA will reduce the effects of viruses on the delta-6-desaturase enzyme while reducing your dietary intake of linoleic acid will reduce the competition with EPA for this enzyme.)

What about flaxseed oil?

Some companies argue that people who need more EPA, such as those who suffer from chronic fatigue syndrome, can get all they need from flaxseed oil, particularly if they are vegetarian (because the oil is derived from the seeds of the flax plant). This is, in my view, a disinguous argument. The omega-3 fatty acid that flaxseed oil provides is alpha-linolenic acid. Looking again at the diagram on page 50 (Figure 5), you will see that alpha-linolenic acid is the dietary precursor of all the long chain omega-3 fatty acids (including EPA). But to get anywhere near EPA down the omega-3 chain, first the alpha-linolenic acid has to be converted into another fatty acid (called octadecatetraenoic acid) which involves the enzyme delta-6-desaturase. However, you will recall that this enzyme can be blocked by various factors, including viruses. Since we are attempting to by-pass this block in chronic fatigue syndrome, it does not make sense to take flaxseed oil.

The ideal formulation

From the information presented in this chapter, we can see that the perfect omega-3 and omega-6 fatty acid formulation to take would be one that contains a combination of:

- Virgin evening primrose oil (as opposed to ordinary refined evening primrose oil that is lacking in free radical-scavenging triterpines)

- Pure EPA

- Zero DHA.

At the time of writing there is only one supplement available on the market that provides this ideal combination. This is VegEPA, available at www.vegepa.com. Each VegEPA capsule contains:

- 100 milligrams (mg) virgin evening primrose oil

- 280 mg pure EPA

- Zero DHA.

As you would expect from our discussion earlier, the capsules are free of any pollutants.

6
The vitamin and mineral cofactors

What are cofactors?

You may have noticed in the preceding chapters that when you take a fatty acid supplement as a natural treatment for chronic fatigue syndrome, there are many enzymes involved in the reactions that have to take place in the body. Some of these include:

- The conversion of the omega-6 fatty acid GLA into dihmo-gamma-linolenic acid. (The enzyme involved is called *elongase*.)

- The conversion of the omega-6 fatty acid dihomo-gamma-linolenic acid into arachidonic acid. (The enzyme involved is called *delta-5-desaturase* – not to be confused with *delta-6-desaturase*.)

- The conversion of dihomo-gamma-linolenic acid and arachidonic acid into different families of eicosanoids.

- The conversion of the omega-3 fatty acid EPA into docosapentaenoic acid (using the enzyme *elongase*). Then the conversion of docosapentaenoic acid into tetra cosapentaenoic acid (using the enzyme *elongase*). Then the conversion of tetracosapentaenoic acid into tetra hexaenoic acid (using the enzyme *delta-6-desaturase*). Then the conversion of tetrahexaenoic acid into DHA (using beta-oxidation).

- The conversion of EPA into different families of eicosanoids.

- The conversion of EPA into interferons. (The enzymes involved include *cyclo-oxygenase* and *lipo-oxygenase*.)

The details in the above list are not particularly important for our purposes. Instead, I want to draw your attention to the many enzymes involved. You can see these at a glance as they are shown in italics. In fact, I have only skimmed the surface in this respect; there are many more involved. For all these enzymes and enzyme-mediated conversions to function properly, small amounts of certain vitamins and minerals need to be present in the body. These are known as cofactors, and their absence makes it difficult for all the reactions to take place properly. So we need to make sure we are not deficient in any of these cofactors.

The most important cofactors

The main vitamins that we need are:

- Folic acid

- Vitamin B_{12}

- Vitamin B_6

- Niacin

- Biotin

- Vitamin C.

These are all B vitamins, apart from the last one (vitamin C). The main minerals (actually trace elements) we need are:

- Zinc

- Selenium

- Magnesium.

If we are deficient in these vitamins, it may be because we are not eating the right foods that are rich in them, or it may be that we are not absorbing the food properly (malabsorption). If you believe that you have an illness that is causing you not to absorb your food properly, then you should see your doctor. Here, I shall assume that you can absorb your intake of these B vitamins, vitamin C, and trace elements.

In general, it is better to obtain these cofactors naturally, in your diet. This means you need to know which foods are rich in each cofactor. This chapter will give you this information. For those of you who prefer to 'play safe' and take vitamin and mineral supplementation, there is a brief section that deals with this at the end of this chapter.

The B vitamins

Folic acid, vitamin B_{12}, vitamin B_6, niacin and biotin are all B vitamins. They are water-soluble vitamins. Being water-soluble, the B vitamins can leach into cooking water and excessive intake from food is rarely dangerous because the B vitamins can be excreted from your body in your urine.

Folic acid

Folic acid is also known as folate and folacin. One of its chemical names is pteroylmonoglutamic acid. Unlike the other B vitamins, folic acid can actually be stored in the liver, and so it is not quite so important to maintain a regular intake of this vitamin. In the United Kingdom, the recommended intake is 200 micrograms per day. A microgram is a millionth of a gram. This is a very small amount.

Good dietary sources of folic acid include:

- Leafy green vegetables

- Beans

- Peas

- Pulses (such as lentils)

- Yeast extract

- Mushrooms

- Nuts

- Whole grains

- Liver

- Certain fortified breakfast cereals.

With this and the other lists of foods given below for each cofactor, the important thing is to make sure you get at least one portion of at least one of the foods in your diet each day. There is really no need to weigh out the food to try to ensure that you are eating the recommended intake. For one thing, the recommended intake can vary between different countries. More importantly, in general the body only needs a small amount of these vitamins and minerals every day. If you are not deficient to begin with, then so long as you are eating something from the lists each day, you should be all right.

For those readers with an interest in medicine, I shall simply note that a deficiency of folic acid can cause megaloblastic or macrocytic anaemia, without going into any further details about what this condition is.

Vitamin B$_{12}$

Vitamin B$_{12}$ consists of a group of molecules which all contain the element cobalt. Collectively they are known as cobalamins, with subtypes including hydroxocobalamin and cyanocobalamin.

Earlier in the book I have explained that certain microbes, notably viruses, appear (at least to me) to lie at the heart of chronic fatigue syndrome. I should not want readers to get the impression, though, that all microbes are bad for us. Far from it. Some microbes are actually good for us and can help supply our bodies with certain nutrients. Vitamin B_{12} is an example where this applies.

Although vitamin B_{12} is not of vegetable origin, in general healthy vegetarians should be able to obtain sufficient quantities from microbes that are to be found in the gastrointestinal tract (particularly the intestines and the mouth). Also, microbial contamination of food will deliver vitamin B_{12} to the human body. Yes, a bit of food contamination is not necessarily a bad thing!

Having said that, there is a theoretical risk that strict vegetarians who eat food that has been irradiated to kill all microbes may eventually become deficient. In healthy individuals, there is enough vitamin B_{12} stored in the liver to last for at least three years. In the United Kingdom, the recommended intake is 1.5 micrograms per day; the corresponding figure is 2 micrograms per day in the United States. (This is just one of many examples in which the United States has set a slightly different recommended daily allowance to that set in the United Kingdom.)

Dietary sources of vitamin B_{12} include:

• Meat

• Milk

• Contamination of food with micro-organisms, mould, faecal matter, insects or insect droppings.

Although milk is a good source, the vitamin may be destroyed by boiling the milk, or adding it to boiling water when making tea or coffee.

A deficiency of vitamin B_{12} can cause megaloblastic or macrocytic anaemia, and prolonged deficiency can lead to subacute combined degeneration of the spinal cord.

Vitamin B_6

Vitamin B_6 is available in food in the forms pyridoxine, pyridoxal and pyridoxamine. These three forms of vitamin B_6 are all active and can be converted to each other. In the United Kingdom, the recommended daily intake is 1.5 micrograms per gram of dietary protein.

Good dietary sources of vitamin B_6 include:

- Whole grains

- Cereals

- Leafy green vegetables

- Eggs

- Meat

- Liver

- Fish

- Pulses

- Fruit

- Green beans.

Deficiency is rare. A deficiency of vitamin B_6 in babies can cause convulsions. Some medications can interact with this vitamin and can thereby produce vitamin B_6 deficiency. They include: isoniazid, hydralazine and penicillamine. A deficiency in adults can lead to anaemia, a smooth and inflamed tongue, lips that are raw with lesions in the corner of the mouth, dermatitis, and fatigue. (Dermatitis is inflammation of the skin. It is essentially the same thing as eczema.)

Niacin

Niacin is also known as nicotinic acid or vitamin B_3. It can be made by the liver from an amino acid called tryptophan; 60 milligrams of dietary tryptophan are converted into 1 milligram of niacin. (One milligram is a thousandth of a gram.) Eggs and cheese are good sources of tryptophan. It tends to be added to many breakfast cereals and to white flour in many countries. (Niacin is lost when wheat is processed to make white flour.) In the United Kingdom, the recommended daily intake is 6.6 milligrams per 1000 kcal dietary energy intake. (One kcal is a kilocalorie, which is one thousand calories. This is a measure of the energy content of food.)

Good dietary sources of niacin include:

• Pulses

• Meat

• Milk

• Nuts

• Liver

• Fish

• Whole grains

• Certain fortified breakfast cereals.

A deficiency of niacin can cause pellagra, in which dermatitis, diarrhoea and dementia occur. Niacin deficiency can occur in people who almost only eat maize (for instance, in some parts of Africa), partly because maize is low in tryptophan and partly because the niacin in maize is present in the form niacytin, which is not active biologically in the same way as ordinary niacin. Niacin deficiency can also occur following treatment with the drug isoniazid. Those who eat a diet that contains a very low level of proteins can also become niacin deficient, as can those who suffer from alcoholism and do not eat properly.

Other causes of niacin deficiency include the carcinoid syndrome and phaeochromocytomas. Carcinoid syndrome is a condition in which patients can suffer from facial and neck blushing, abdominal pains and watery diarrhoea which keeps recurring, as well as some heart problems. It can result from a particular type of growth in the bowels, called carcinoid tumours, which have spread to the liver.

These tumours secrete the transmitter serotonin, which causes the diarrhoea. (Patients with chronic fatigue syndrome who have been prescribed SSRI antidepressants may also suffer from diarrhoea for the same reason. SSRI stands for selective serotonin re-uptake inhibitor. These antidepressants raise the levels of serotonin. A list of the main SSRI and SSRI-related antidepressants is given in Chapter 8, on pages 124-125.)

Phaeochromocytomas are tumours that arise usually in the adrenal glands. (The adrenal glands are two glands that lie just above the kidneys.) They secrete noradrenaline (also known as norepinephrine) and adrenaline (epinephrine) into the circulation.

Biotin

Biotin is also known as coenzyme R, vitamin H and, originally, the anti-egg white injury factor. In the United Kingdom, the recommended intake is between 10 and 200 micrograms per day, while in the United States the corresponding recommended intake range is between 30 and 100 micrograms per day.

Good dietary sources of biotin include:

- Nuts

- Fruit

- Whole, brown rice

- Yeast

- Cooked eggs

- Cereals

- Liver.

A deficiency of biotin can occur in those who eat a lot of raw eggs, owing to the fact that raw egg white protein contains a protein (avidin) that acts to prevent absorption of biotin; this protein is destroyed by cooking eggs. If a mother is not well-fed, then her breast milk may be very low in biotin, which can cause dermatitis in her baby.

In adults, taking biotin can help rejuvenate the hair follicles. In other words, if you are beginning to lose hair, sometimes taking biotin can help your hair follicles to start growing thicker hair again. If, in addition, you take a fatty acid supplement that contains virgin evening primrose oil and pure EPA, then you are feeding your hair follicles with excellent nutrients. (One gentleman of my acquaintance started to take a fatty acid supplement that contains virgin evening primrose oil and pure EPA every day. Within eight weeks his hair had started to change from being dry and wiry into a luscious growth of a soft and glossier covering of his scalp. His barber was pleasantly surprised. Incidentally, his skin also changed. When he started the supplement he could have passed for a sixty-year-old. Now he looks as if he is in his forties.)

Vitamin C

Vitamin C is also known as ascorbic acid or ascorbate and is water-soluble. Unlike most other mammals, unfortunately human bodies cannot make their own vitamin C and so we must obtain this important antioxidant in our diets. In the United Kingdom, the recommended daily intake is 40 milligrams, while the corresponding figure in the United States is 60 milligrams. The late Linus Pauling (winner of two Nobel prizes) recommended much higher doses, although if there is any impairment of kidney function, then a very high dose can lead to the formation of kidney stones. Linus Pauling argued that the government nutrition bodies were being too conservative. By looking at the amount of vitamin C that an average adult gorilla eats each day in the wild, and then extrapolating back to the average human body weight, he suggested that we need well over a gram of this vitamin each day.

Good dietary sources of vitamin C include:

- Fruit – such as citrus fruits, fresh strawberries, cantaloupe, pineapples and guava

- Vegetables – such as broccoli, Brussels sprouts, tomatoes, potatoes, spinach, kale, green peppers, cabbage and turnips

- Fresh milk.

Vitamin C is readily leached out of vegetables that are being cooked in water. Cooking also oxidizes the vitamin, as does exposure to alkalis or copper. The vitamin C content of potatoes gradually diminishes with storage of this vegetable. Deficiency of vitamin C sometimes occurs in infants who are fed boiled milk. A deficiency of vitamin C can cause scurvy, in which at first there may be weakness and muscle pains, followed by more classical sign in which the gums bleed, teeth become loose, wounds do not heal properly, and there is bleeding under the skin. Anaemia is also likely, as vitamin C is needed to help with the absorption of iron from the diet.

The trace elements

Trace elements are mineral elements that are required in trace amounts in the diet for the maintenance of good health. Zinc, selenium and magnesium are all trace elements that have to be obtained by dietary means.

Zinc

Zinc can help wound healing, prostate problems and infertility. It can help promote mental alertness. In the United Kingdom, the recommended daily intake is 9.5 milligrams for men and 7 milligrams for women.

Good dietary sources of zinc include:

- Meat

- Wholegrain products

- Pulses

• Yeast

• Pumpkin seeds.

Clinically, zinc deficiency may cause white spots under the fingernails and poor healing of wounds. With severe zinc deficiency, there may be loss of hair, night blindness, and impairment of taste and smell.

Selenium

Selenium acts as an antioxidant in conjunction with vitamin E. It can help return a youthful elasticity to tissues, and alleviate some of the effects of the menopause such as hot flushes. In the United Kingdom, the recommended intake of selenium is 60 micrograms per day.

Good dietary sources of selenium include:

• Meat

• Wholegrain products

• Fish

• Vegetables.

In some countries, such as the United States and Canada, the soil is relatively rich in selenium, so that the bread made there contains sufficient quantities. However, European wheat is rather impoverished in this respect, while the soil in parts of China has very low levels of this trace element.

Severe selenium deficiency can cause a potentially fatal heart disease (cardiomyopathy) known as Keshan disease; this sometime occurs in those parts of China where the population depends on crops grown on selenium deficient soil. It is not known whether there are any direct clinical effects from mild selenium deficiency, other than adverse effects on making fatty acids.

Magnesium

Magnesium occurs as part of the green chlorophyll pigment of plants.

It helps promote a healthy cardiovascular system and is involved in calcium metabolism. Its levels in the human body can become depleted by alcohol.

Good dietary sources of magnesium include:

- Vegetables – particularly fresh green ones and corn

- Pulses

- Fruit – including apples.

A severe deficiency, for example as a result of alcoholism, can cause seizures.

Supplements

It is best to obtain the above cofactors (the B vitamins, vitamin C, and the trace elements) from your diet, by ensuring that your daily food intake includes at least one of the foodstuffs from the list for each cofactor. However, there may be a problem in adhering to such a regime. For example, you may be too busy to be able to find the time to eat a proper suitably varied diet. Or you may find that you are sometimes too tired to prepare such meals. In such cases, it is better to take a supplement rather than miss out altogether on these cofactors.

For the B vitamins, there are vitamin B complex supplements available, while vitamin C supplements (both tablets that are swallowed and tablets and powder preparations that are dissolved in water) can also be readily bought over-the-counter in chemists (pharmacies) and supermarkets. To be on the safe side and make sure you do not miss out on any of these vitamins, you could consider taking a multivitamin supplement. If choosing a multivitamin, you should check that it does deliver all the B vitamins mentioned above. In general, it is a good idea to take just the stated dose. In other words, unless you have carefully researched the doses and know why you want to take a high dose of a certain vitamin, then it is safest to stay within the Recommended Daily Allowances for each vitamin. (Some people are happy to take higher doses of vitamin C, for example, but in such cases they should ensure they do not suffer from kidney disease, in order that kidney stones are not formed.)

A similar set of considerations applies to the choice of supplements of trace elements. Buying multimineral supplements that contain zinc, selenium and magnesium is often cheaper than purchasing separate supplements for each of these three trace elements. In the cases of zinc and selenium, I would strongly recommend that you stay within the Recommended Daily Allowances for each trace element. It is possible to suffer from the effects of toxicity if too much zinc or selenium is taken each day.

Finally, there are some preparations available that are combined multivitamin and multimineral supplements. So long as they contain all the cofactors mentioned in this chapter, then it is absolutely fine to take these at the stated dose.

7

Other benefits from taking fatty acids

There are a number of known side-effects from taking an omega-3 and omega-6 fatty acid supplement but none that are seriously adverse and many that are wholly beneficial. I will examine them in this chapter.

The only side effect that might be regarded as adverse is a slight loosening of the bowel contents. This may occur with a dose of eight VegEPA capsules daily. However, this is actually a good thing because if the passage of material speeds up in your gut, then there is less time for toxins to be absorbed into your system. Some scientists think that as a result you might reduce your risks of getting bowel cancer. (You can also speed things up by ensuring you have a lot of fibre in your diet. A good way to do this is to choose unrefined products over refined products. For example, wholemeal flour and bread are better than white flour and bread. Again, brown rice is better than white rice.)

The other 'side-effects' of a supplement containing pure EPA and virgin evening primrose oil are also good for us. In fact, they are so beneficial that, in general, almost everyone can benefit from taking such a supplement daily (albeit at a lower dose of, say, four VegEPA capsules daily for those who do not suffer from chronic fatigue syndrome or depression). The only slight caution is in respect of those who are taking a blood-thinning drug such as warfarin or heparin – this is explained below in the section entitled 'Cardiovascular system'. In fact, although I have never suffered from either chronic fatigue syndrome or depression, I take eight capsules daily, as four each morning and four each evening, with food.

Mood and combating depression

Pure EPA (without any DHA) acts as a powerful, yet safe, mood elevating substance. In fact, so good is pure EPA in doing this that it has actually been found to have antidepressant actions in severe depression.

Evidence from epidemiology

In 1998, Joe Hibbeln, from the National Institutes of Health in Maryland, in the United States, published a letter in The Lancet in which he pointed out that when he had looked at data for nine countries comparing the annual rate of depression with the annual apparent fish consumption (calculated by fish catch plus imports minus exports), there was a negative relationship between these. On the one hand, countries such as New Zealand, West Germany (before the fall of the Berlin Wall) and Canada were found to have high rates of depression of around five to six cases per 100 adults, but low apparent fish consumption of less than 50 pounds (23 kilograms) per person. On the other hand, Japan was found to have an annual rate of depression of less than 0.13 cases per 100 adults, but a high apparent fish consumption of almost 150 pounds (68 kilograms) per person.

In 1993, Michael Maes' team published an important paper in the *American Journal of Psychiatry* based on national data for Belgium for the period 1979 to 1987. It showed that there was a seasonal variation in the rate of violent suicide. In a further paper by the same group (De Vriese and colleagues, 2004), Professor Maes' team showed that this seasonal variation in the rate of violent suicide is negatively related to the seasonal variation in the level of EPA.

An important reason why the level of EPA in the body can vary is because the level of EPA in the diet often undergoes a seasonal variation. For example, if cows are fed on pasture, then their milk is likely to contain EPA. If, during the autumn and winter months, they are no longer fed on grass, but instead are grain-fed, then their milk will no longer contain any EPA at that time of year. The same applies to the level of EPA in dairy products such as butter, and in meat such as beef and lamb. (In general, the traditional practices of animal husbandry in which cattle, lambs and sheep are allowed to graze openly on pastures all year round are the best for our diet.)

Taken together, both these sets of studies indicate a link between low levels of EPA and the occurrence of depression or suicide.

Evidence from biochemistry

There is strong and consistent evidence that the levels of omega-3 long-chain polyunsaturated fatty acids, particularly EPA, are reduced in the plasma and red blood cell membranes of depressed patients. The interested reader can obtain full details from my chapter entitled 'Lipids, eicosapentaenoic acid, and depression' in the book *Nutrients, Stress, Medical Disorders* due to be published in 2004 or early 2005.

Clinical studies of depression

In a detailed case report published in 2001 in the *International Journal of Clinical Practice* and in 2002 in *Archives of General Psychiatry*, my colleagues and I published evidence for the first time that a young man with severe, intractable depression that had not previously responded to ordinary psychiatric drug treatment (including powerful modern antidepressants and lithium) fully recovered when he was given pure EPA.

At the time of writing, three major trials have been published in which patients with depression have been treated successfully with EPA. For example, Nehmets and colleagues carried out a trial in Israel in which they showed that a supplement of 2 grams of pure (ethyl-) EPA per day caused a striking reduction in depression in just four weeks. Two grams of pure (ethyl-) EPA per day can be obtained by taking between seven and eight VegEPA capsules per day. (The EPA in VegEPA is also in the pure (ethyl) form, with no DHA being present. An advantage of this product is that it also contains virgin evening primrose oil.)

Sleep

EPA is converted into natural sleep mediators. After a few days to a few weeks of taking pure EPA (without any DHA), even people who do not suffer from chronic fatigue syndrome find that they experience sleep that is much deeper and much more refreshing than they might be used to. From personal experience, the best description I can think of to describe just how pleasant this sleep is (and I had never had problems sleeping during my adult life prior to starting to take EPA) is a verse from the Wisdom literature to be found in the Bible in Proverbs chapter 3 verse 24:

> Yea, thou shalt lie down,
> And thy sleep shall be sweet.

Energy

Even in those who have never suffered from chronic fatigue syndrome, regular intake of an omega-3 and omega-6 fatty acid supplement is associated with increased energy levels. Part of this may be by virtue of the improved more refreshing sleep that they enjoy. There are also other reasons for the improved energy, including the fact that the body's cells and tissues are now able to make sufficient quantities of different eicosanoid families (see Chapter 4) from virgin evening primrose oil and pure EPA. The body now has at its disposal a full complement of stress-busting substances within the context of an immune system that is geared up and finely tuned, ready for action against any potential microbial invader.

Concentration and thinking

Whether or not a person is suffering from chronic fatigue syndrome to begin with, they are likely to find that their concentration and general thinking ability is much improved within weeks of starting a supplement containing pure EPA (without DHA) and virgin evening primrose oil.

I know of one child who had previously suffered from the features of attention-deficit hyperactivity disorder, being very restless, fidgety and unable to settle down and concentrate. Within just three months of taking an omega-3 and omega-6 fatty acid supplement, all these problems disappeared. What was equally astonishing to his mother was that he suddenly started showing a strong interest in books. Rather than sit in front of the television all evening, he now preferred to read. Before this particular study, I had thought that the malign influence of television was to blame for the general reduction in reading skills and reading for pleasure that we see in children (particularly boys) these days. I have had to revise my opinion in light of this and other examples. It now seems to me that perhaps children (and adults) find it easier and more enjoyable to read when they have higher levels of omega-3 and omega-6 fatty acids.

Cardiovascular system

Eskimo diet

In the 1950s, Dr Hugh Sinclair of Oxford University, mentor to Professor David Horrobin (who in turn was one of my mentors), discovered that the Inuit did not suffer from anywhere near as much heart disease and high blood pressure as those living in Western countries, in spite of the fact that they ate large amounts of 'animal fats' such as fish and seals. Clinically, one good way of looking at how furred up the arteries are is to look at the eyes. The coloured part of the eye, the iris, which surrounds the black pupil in the middle, gradually starts to develop an outer annular whitish ring as hardening of the arteries and deposition of fat take place in the arteries of the body. Surprisingly, Sinclair found that this annulus (known as an *arcus senilis*) did not seem to occur in the Inuit who were eating their traditional Eskimo diet, even when the individuals concerned were of advanced years. This finding furnished further evidence of a healthy cardiovascular system.

Although Hugh Sinclair attributed this healthy state of affairs to the high dietary intake by the Inuit of omega-3 fatty acids, at first this explanation was rejected by some in the medical establishment, who argued instead that what Sinclair had discovered were the effects of a special genetic adaptation that had occurred during the many centuries that this population had spent genetically isolated from other human   gene pools. In other words, this argument attributed the resistance of the Inuit to cardiovascular disease to their genes.

Evidence supporting Hugh Sinclair's contention came to light when epidemiological studies were carried out of Inuit communities who had emigrated to Canada. When members of this population moved from their traditional high-omega-3 Eskimo diet to a Western diet, their levels of cardiovascular disease, including heart attacks and thrombotic strokes, rose to match that in the more indigenous Western populations around them. In fact, other diseases which had also appeared to be relatively uncommon in those Inuit on a high-omega-3 diet also rose to match those of people in the West generally once the Inuit changed their diets to a very low-omega-3 typical Western diet. These diseases included arthritis and other joint problems, diabetes and its complications such as neuropathy (nerve damage), and skin diseases such as eczema.

Benefits of high EPA

In addition to examining their eyes, Hugh Sinclair carried out another test that was fairly easy to perform in the Eskimo populations of Greenland without ready recourse to advanced laboratories and hospitals. This was to measure how quickly the blood clotted – in other words, how 'thin' the blood was – for the individuals he saw. What he found was that bleeding time in the Inuit was much longer than in people on typical non-omega-3-rich diets.

Normally, if we cut ourselves, after a couple of minutes or so the cut stops bleeding as the previously oozing blood starts to clot and form a solid barrier. This is generally a useful thing but under certain circumstances a propensity for the blood to clot within a couple of minutes can be a distinct disadvantage. Here are three important examples. The first is the tendency for a blood clot to form in the blood vessels (deep veins) of the calf muscles of the lower leg following prolonged periods of inactivity of the legs, as may occur during a long-haul flight or even a long coach journey. This may cause tenderness of the calf and swelling of the lower leg. The person may also start to suffer from a slight fever. On reaching their destination, the traveller will get up from their cramped sitting position and may dislodge the clot (or thrombus) or cause smaller clots to break off. In turn, these clots may then travel up the veins of the body and, via the right-side of the heart, into the major vessels in the lungs, where they may lodge. This is known as pulmonary embolism. The patient may become breathless, suffer from chest pain, find there is blood in their spit (sputum), become dizzy and faint. Their temperature and heart rate may rise, their blood pressure may fall, and they may develop bluish lips. In the case of large clots lodging in the lungs, the patient may die. Since this condition starts with the formation of a clot or thrombus in deep veins, it is known as deep-vein thrombosis, or DVT for short. The second example relates to when a clot forms in one of the coronary arteries that supplies the heart with blood. This means that the part of the heart tissue that is deprived of a blood supply may start to die – this is a 'heart attack'. My final example relates to the occurrence of a clot in one of the blood vessels of the brain. If this happens, then the blood supply to part of the brain is cut off, leading to damage and possible death of some brain tissue. This is a stroke (or, more accurately, a thrombotic stroke).

So, if the blood is 'thinner' and less likely to clot as a result of a high intake of EPA, then there is clearly a reduced risk of suffering from a deep-vein thrombosis, or from pulmonary embolism, a heart attack or a thrombotic stroke.

If you have suffered from a deep-vein thrombosis, or from pulmonary embolism, a heart attack or a thrombotic stroke, then as part of your medical treatment you may be put on a blood thinning medicine. Initially this is often heparin, in the form of injections, while later, after discharge from hospital, it is likely to be warfarin, acenocoumarol or phenindione in the form of tablets. (Warfarin is also used as rat poison, thinning rats' blood to such a degree that they bleed uncontrollably.) In 2005, a new blood thinning drug called ximelagastran (Exanta) is being introduced. If you are on such medication, then you should consult your doctor if you decide to start taking a supplement of omega-3 fatty acids. This is so that the doctor can make any necessary adjustments to your blood thinning drugs, just in case your blood thins noticeably further as a result of taking the supplement. In practice, it is worth pointing out that a fatty acid supplement is unlikely to thin your blood to such an extent as to be noticeable. I have been taking eight VegEPA capsules daily for several months, purely for the health benefits they give me, and all I have noticed are these benefits, without any bleeding problems at all; my blood does take longer to clot, which is a good thing, but I have not noticed any greater tendency to bruise.

Atrial fibrillation

The heart has four chambers, the two upper 'atria' and the lower two 'ventricles'. In a healthy heart the atria pump blood into the ventricles. However, in certain conditions, the upper atria, instead of pumping blood into the lower ventricles in a purposeful rhythmic manner, lose their rhythm and just seem almost to quiver, so that the heart is not as effective a pump as it should be. This condition is known as atrial fibrillation. Conditions that can cause it include ischaemic heart disease (in which the heart is deprived of its own blood supply, such as following a 'heart attack'), problems with certain heart valves, rheumatic heart disease, high blood pressure, overactive thyroid or 'hyperthyroidism' (thyrotoxicosis), heart surgery and pulmonary embolism (blood clots in the vessels of the lungs).

　　　Dr Dariush Mozaffarian, from Brigham and Women's Hospital and Harvard Medical School in Boston, Massachusetts, and colleagues, assessed 4,815 adults aged 65 years or older in 1989 and 1990. These assessments included dietary details. During a 12-year follow-up period, during which these subjects had annual heart tracings (electrocardiograms), there were 980 cases of atrial fibrillation.

Analysis of the data showed that the higher the intake of tuna, or other broiled or baked fish, the lower the rate of atrial fibrillation. In other words, a high intake of omega-3 fatty acids is associated with a reduced risk of atrial fibrillation. These results were published in 2004 in the journal *Circulation*.

Joints

Arthritis afflicts increasing numbers of people as we collectively get older. It is a condition in which there is inflammation of one or more of the joints in the body. This manifests as pain, swelling, redness, stiffness and warmth of the joint or joints. The sufferer might also sometimes be feverish. A major form of arthritis is osteoarthritis, in which there is degeneration of the protective cartilage around the ends of two bones that meet in the joint. The amount of the nourishing and cushioning fluid in the joint (known as synovial fluid) is also diminished as the osteoarthritis progresses. The resulting wearing action of one bone on the other, without sufficient intervening cartilage and synovial fluid, can cause excruciating pain.

Osteoarthritis and some cases of other types of arthritis (such as rheumatoid arthritis) are helped by taking a combination of EPA and virgin evening primrose oil. The EPA helps restore the functioning of the synovial fluid of the joints, while a particularly important helpful component of virgin evening primrose oil is the family of triterpines that were described briefly in Chapter 5.

A suitable starting dose for arthritis would be between four and eight VegEPA capsules daily, depending on the severity of the joint problems.

Body weight

If you are not very depressed or very underweight to begin with, then you need not worry that taking a supplement such as VegEPA may cause an increase in your body weight. In fact, if anything, if you are overweight to begin with, you may well notice that you start to become slimmer. This is partly because the fatty acids in this supplement have an effect on the brain that causes the body to feel as if it has eaten enough sooner than it would if you were not taking the supplement.

Skin, hair and nails

Within a few weeks of starting a fatty acid supplement containing pure EPA and virgin evening primrose oil, most people (whether or not they have been suffering from chronic fatigue syndrome) begin to notice a striking improvement in their skin, hair and nails.

Those who have been suffering from dry skin notice that their skin is no longer dry but is being moisturized from the inside in a totally natural way. If they suffered from dry lips and/or a dry mouth, they find that these conditions also clear up, perhaps for the first time in many years. I have found that patients' skin looks so much better that often their partners insist that they too wish to start taking the supplement in order to benefit from the same natural, more youthful looking skin that it causes. There is absolutely no harm in doing this (so long as the person checks first with their doctor if they are taking a blood thinning drug such as warfarin or heparin). In fact, given the many benefits of EPA and virgin evening primrose oil, it could be argued that there is a case for actively encouraging people to take such a supplement.

In addition to making your skin look much better and more youthful, omega-3 and omega-6 fatty acid supplements help keep your hair glossy and better-looking. This is particularly noticeable if you previously suffered from dry hair, perhaps with split ends. I am reminded of a letter I received in 2004 from a woman who had suffered from chronic fatigue syndrome for many years. After just two months she reported that:

> I am still taking the VegEPA. I have found a big improvement in [my] skin, my hair has gone very shiny... and I have managed a gradual return to work.

EPA combined with virgin evening primrose oil is also wonderfully good for your nails. Many people notice that, after the first three months, their nails are the best they can ever remember. Again, this is particularly noticeable if they were previously dry and brittle or unduly soft.

8

Treating chronic fatigue syndrome naturally

In this, the final chapter, we shall go through some practical issues related to the natural treatment of chronic fatigue syndrome. We shall look at the sort of medical assessment that a patient needs. Then we shall consider the ways to tell if you are deficient in omega-3 and omega-6 fatty acids. Next, we shall look at issues relating to omega-3 and omega-6 fatty acid supplementation, changes in diet, exercise and complementary therapies.

The medical assessment

I am an advocate of carrying out a very thorough medical assessment of patients who are suspected of having chronic fatigue syndrome. There are four aspects to such an assessment, which altogether might easily last two hours:

- Clinical history

- Mental state examination

- Physical examination

- Laboratory investigations.

During the whole process the doctor looks for evidence that there is another cause for the patient's symptoms other than chronic fatigue syndrome. It is somewhat akin to a good 'Whodunnit', in which the doctor plays the role of the detective. (I have sometimes wondered whether my professional practice is related to my love of Agatha Christie and Colin Dexter.)

Clinical history

I always take a very detailed clinical history from new patients referred to me for the first time. I feel it is important to be patient and allow the patient to tell his or her account of the development of the illness in their own time. I also try to interview a relative if that is appropriate, for example the spouse of an adult patient or one or both parents of an adolescent patient. In such cases, it is useful to see both the patient and their relative (or other close friend) on their own. Talking to each individually without the presence of the other means that they each feel less inhibited about discussing matters that might seem a little embarrassing or private. The clinical history can be a very strong indicator of:

- Contributing causes or precipitants of the chronic fatigue syndrome

- How deficient in fatty acids the patient is (see below)

- Evidence of any other illness that might be presenting with chronic fatigue syndrome-like symptoms.

Mental state examination

The mental state examination refers to a specialized interview that those doctors who specialize in psychiatry learn to carry out. It is a way of assessing the workings of the mind of the patient, including a person's mood, intellectual functioning, memory and personality. Is he or she depressed, for example, and, if so, to what degree?

After years of training it is possible to investigate a patient's mental state in a detailed but considerate way without causing offence. Often, if a patient is feeling low, say, they find it cathartic to be able to talk to a doctor about this.

Physical examination

It is important that the doctor carries out a thorough physical examination. Already, from the clinical history taking and the mental state examination the conscientious doctor will have clues as to which particular 'organic' diseases (other than chronic fatigue syndrome) may be present. These possible diagnoses are listed on page xxx. A detailed physical examination allows the doctor to obtain more evidence which might clinch the diagnosis.

Laboratory investigations

If a doctor suspects that their patient may be suffering from a certain illness (other than chronic fatigue syndrome), they may order some extra investigations. Fukuda and colleagues, in their revised CDC criteria for chronic fatigue syndrome, which we described in Chapter 2, recommend that the following minimum battery of laboratory screening tests should be carried out for all new referrals:

- Full blood count, including a white cell (leukocyte) differential

- Erythrocyte sedimentation rate (ESR)

- Alanine aminotransferase

- Total protein

- Albumin

- Globulin

- Alkaline phosphatase

- Calcium

- Phosphorus

- Glucose

- Blood urea nitrogen

- Electrolytes

- Creatinine

- Thyroid stimulating hormone

- Urine tests.

All but the last of these investigations are carried out on a blood sample. In addition, there are other tests that can be carried out which neither confirm nor exclude the diagnosis of chronic fatigue syndrome. Examples include carrying out blood serological studies. These are specialized tests looking for evidence of infection. The particular infections looked for are those caused by the following organisms:

- Epstein-Barr virus (which causes glandular fever and Burkitt's lymphoma)

- Retroviruses (which can cause AIDS, myelopathy, and certain forms of lymphoma and leukaemia)

- Human herpesvirus 6 (which can cause meningitis and encephalitis)

- Enteroviruses (which can cause meningitis, encephalitis, heart disease, muscle disease, and diseases of the hand, foot and mouth)

- Candida albicans (which can cause oral and vaginal thrush).

Other illnesses

There are many other illnesses that may present with symptoms similar to those that occur in chronic fatigue syndrome. According to the CDC, some of the key ones, which the whole process of clinical history taking, mental state examination, physical examination and laboratory investigations is aimed at detecting, include:

- Untreated hypothyroidism

- Sleep apnoea (in which the airway is blocked during sleep – the interruption of breathing awakens the person, often only briefly, before they fall asleep again and the whole cycle repeats itself)

- Narcolepsy (in which the person is overcome with episodes of irresistible sleep during what should be waking hours)

- Side-effects of medication

- Previously treated cancer

- Unresolved cases of hepatitis B or C virus infection

- Depression

- Bipolar disorder

- Schizophrenia

- Dementia

- Anorexia nervosa

- Bulimia nervosa

- Alcohol abuse up to two years before the onset of the chronic fatigue

- Drug abuse up to two years before the onset of the chronic fatigue

- Severe obesity.

Fatty acid deficiency

Having carried out a thorough medical assessment, excluded the possibility of another illness, and therefore confirmed the working clinical diagnosis of chronic fatigue syndrome, the next thing I do is to assess the level of fatty acid deficiency. There are two ways of doing this. The method I prefer is to look for clinical features of fatty acid deficiency. The other way is to take a blood sample for measurement of the levels of omega-3 and omega-6 fatty acids in the membranes of the red blood cells.

Clinical features

There are several features that can be related to fatty acid deficiency. These include:

- Dry hair

- Problems with the nails – soft or brittle, for example

- Skin problems – dryness, roughness, eczema, psoriasis

- Suffering from dry lips for much of the day

- Suffering from a dry mouth for much of the day

- Usually feeling more thirsty than would be expected by the circumstances

- Poor sleep

- Having hands that become particularly cold or change colour sometimes, for example in winter

- Having feet that become particularly cold or change colour sometimes, for example in winter

- Needing to pass water more often than is usual for people of the same age

- Suffering from asthma, hayfever or other allergies.

Blood testing

Some specialized centres offer the facility to assess directly the level of omega-3 and omega-6 fatty acids in the membranes of red blood cells. We have seen earlier in this book why this is considered to be a good indicator of the state of the fatty acids in the membranes of organs such as the brain.

Typical normal reference ranges for some of the omega-3 and omega-6 fatty acids are now listed. This means that if the level measured is below the lower end of the range for that particular fatty acid, then there is a deficiency of it in the body. These figures are a guide only; in practice, if the laboratory offers a set of reference ranges, they should be used in preference to the ones listed here. Note that the figures are given as micromoles per litre. A mole, in this context, is a scientific measure referring to the mass (weight) of a substance that contains a certain specified number of molecules (or atoms) of that substance. For example, one mole of the commonest form of the element carbon, known as carbon-12, has a mass of exactly 12 grams. A micromole is one millionth of a mole. So a micromole of carbon-12 has a mass of 12 micrograms.

For the omega-6 fatty acids, typical normal reference ranges are as follows:

- Linoleic acid: 30 to 76 micromoles per litre

- GLA: 0.7 to 2.5 micromoles per litre

- DGLA: 5.0 to 9.7 micromoles per litre

- Arachidonic acid: 28 to 70 micromoles per litre.

For the omega-3 fatty acids, typical normal reference ranges are as follows:

- Alpha-linolenic acid: 2.2 to 5.9 micromoles per litre

- EPA: 2.1 to 7.4 micromoles per litre.

Supplementation

For the reasons given in Chapter 5, the best omega-3 and omega-6 fatty acid supplement to take is one that contains a combination of pure EPA and virgin evening primrose oil (with preferably no DHA whatsoever). The one supplement currently available to the general public that fulfils these criteria is VegEPA. This can be obtained from the web site www.vegepa.com.

A good dose to start with is eight of these capsules daily, taken as four each morning and four each evening, preferably with food. The capsules are fairly small and easy to swallow. If swallowing is too difficult for any reason, then the capsules can be crunched in the mouth and the contents swallowed. It is even possible to cut open the vegetarian capsule shells and squeeze the contents into some fruit juice or into some yoghurt.

It can take around three months for the full benefits to start to become apparent. Once improvement starts to occur, it is worth continuing with the treatment. The dose of eight capsules daily is preferable, but if for any reason you want to take a reduced dosage, then the eight capsules can gradually be cut to six or even four daily, over a period of another three months. In the case of children between the ages of eight and 14 years, the adult doses should be halved.

In the unlikely event that no benefits have been noticed at all after three months, it may be worth having the special red blood cell membrane fatty acid test. This will show whether or not the EPA and omega-6 levels are in the normal range. If they are still rather low (particularly the EPA on the omega-3 side), in spite of eight capsules daily, then there are several things you can do.

First, ensure you are getting enough of the cofactors described in Chapter 6 (several B vitamins, vitamin C, zinc, selenium and magnesium). A good way of doing this is to ensure that your diet is adequate in these vitamins and trace elements; further details of foods rich in these cofactors are given in that chapter. Another way of getting enough cofactors is to take vitamin and mineral supplements. Again, there are further details in Chapter 6.

Second, you may be under too much stress in your daily life.

This could be caused by work colleagues, financial problems, relationship difficulties, concern about relatives, or a host of other reasons. Unfortunately, long-running raised stress levels can raise the levels of stress hormones such as cortisol, which in turn inhibit the proper functioning of the enzyme delta-6-desaturase. This enzyme is involved in the conversion of EPA into DHA, and so it is good to try to reduce the levels of stress in your life. Good stress-busters include exercise and certain complementary therapies (see below), as well as altering the way you think about the things that make you feel stressed. If it comes to the worst, it may be worth making some major lifestyle changes to make your life less stressful.

The third thing you can do is temporarily raise your intake of the supplement to nine or ten capsules daily. After three months, you can come back down to eight capsules per day.

Caffeine, alcohol and smoking

It is possible that caffeine, alcohol and nicotine may inhibit the action of the enzyme delta-6-desaturase. If possible, you should therefore try to reduce your intake of caffeine-containing drinks, such as coffee, cola drinks and tea. If you drink heavily, it would be better to reduce your alcohol consumption to only a moderate amount.

As for nicotine, there is no question that it is extremely bad for your health to smoke. If you are a smoker, you should make every effort to give up. Nowadays there are many aids to stopping smoking. If you need help, just ask your family doctor.

Diet

Cofactors

As discussed in Chapter 6, it is important to eat a healthy diet that is rich in the following cofactors:

- Folic acid

- Vitamin B_{12}

- Vitamin B_6

- Niacin

- Biotin

- Vitamin C

- Zinc

- Selenium

- Magnesium.

You should go through each of these cofactors in turn, and check that you are regularly eating at least one of the foodstuffs that are a good source of each one. (The relevant lists are given in Chapter 6.)

Cofactor supplements

Recently, a very safe multivitamin/multimineral preparation has become available that contains only the particular cofactors mentioned in this chapter and in Chapter 6, and only in doses less than the recommended daily allowances. It is called VegeCO, and is specifically for adults (available from www.vegpa.com). Each VegeCO tablet contains:

Folic acid	100 micrograms
Vitamin B_{12}	0.75 micrograms
Vitamin B_6	0.5 milligrams
Niacin	6 milligrams
Biotin	10 micrograms
Vitamin C	20 milligrams

Zinc	3.5 milligrams
Selenium	30 micrograms
Magnesium	200 micrograms

It is perfectly safe for an adult to take one VegeCO tablet daily.

For children, the equivalent preparation is called mini VegeCO. Each mini VegeCO tablet contains:

Folic acid	10 micrograms
Vitamin B_{12}	0.075 micrograms
Vitamin B_6	0.05 milligrams
Niacin	0.6 milligrams
Biotin	1 microgram
Vitamin C	20 milligrams
Zinc	0.35 milligrams
Selenium	3 micrograms
Magnesium	20 micrograms

Children aged over 12 years can safely take two mini VegeCO tablets daily. (The outer shell of VegeCO and mini VgeCO is vegetarian and so is free of gelatine. Instead it is made from tapioca, which is a cassava root starch.)

Frying food

If you do have to fry anything – and it is far better to avoid frying food at all because the process heats food to such a degree it destroys essential nutrients in the food – then use a small amount of virgin olive oil, which is rich in monounsaturates (making up between 55% and 85% of the oil), but only about 9% of which is linoleic acid.

Manufactured trans fats

When making margarine, vegetable oils are industrially changed to turn them into solids at room temperature. This process is known as hydrogenation, and the result is hydrogenated vegetable fat. Unfortunately, the industrial processes involved cause the fatty acids in the vegetable oil to be turned into strange molecules called trans fats. (The trans in this name refers to a special type of chemical bond in the molecules called trans bonds.)

When ingested, the body treats the trans fats as if they were ordinary naturally occurring fatty acids. This causes at least two sets of profound problems for our health.

First, trans fats inhibit the action of the enzyme delta-6-desaturase. As explained below in the section on cortisol, this means that it becomes more difficult for the body to produce DHA (from EPA). In addition, it also means it is more difficult for the body to produce EPA, DGLA and AA from the dietary fatty acid precursors; this should not be a problem, though, if you are taking a supplement containing pure EPA and virgin evening primrose oil, as you can then produce your own DGLA and AA from the virgin evening primrose oil.

The second problem is that the cells of our body, including those of the brain, unfortunately incorporate the trans fats into their membranes. This makes the membranes very inflexible. In turn, membrane receptors do not work properly and signals do not pass properly between cells. This includes problems with signals passing between brain cells.

The best policy is to remove trans fats from your diet and to put yourself on a high pure EPA and virgin evening primrose oil supplement. But which 'foods' contain these artificial trans fats? Unfortunately, the answer is processed foodstuffs that contain hydrogenated fat, including:

- Margarine

- Pastries

- Most biscuits (unless made with pure butter)

- Most cakes (unless made with pure butter)

- Most pies

- Pre-packed sachets of drinking chocolate and of some coffee preparations.

If you look carefully at the ingredients list on the products you buy, you should be able to avoid most sources.

Butter is an excellent alternative to margarine. It is particularly good to go for a brand of butter that is derived from cows that never eat concentrated feedstock or get confined to sheds. An excellent brand that is widely available is Anchor Butter, from New Zealand. The cows for Anchor Butter roam free and eat fresh green grass all year round. As a result, this particular brand of butter should also contain some EPA (unlike butter from grain-fed cows).

Fried foods

Frying is generally bad for you, as it harms the omega-3 fatty acids in foods such as fish, to say nothing of the production of poisons such as acrylamide. In the study by Dr Dariush Mozaffarian and colleague, published in 2004 and described in the previous chapter, in which a diet rich in fish containing omega-3 fatty acids was found to reduce the risk of atrial fibrillation, another finding was that this protective effect of dietary fish did not apply to fish that had been fried.

Suitable alternatives to frying are steaming or lightly grilling your food. You are less likely to create acrylamide by steaming your food, and both steaming and light grilling are less likely than frying to harm the omega-3 fatty acids in your food.

Sugar

Ordinary sugar (or sucrose), particularly white sugar, can cause harm to the body in many ways. One of these relates to its effects on our energy levels. After the immediate rush that occurs following a meal or drink that contains added sugar, your energy levels may actually feel as if they have diminished, as your body tries hard to mop up all the extra sugar by pouring out insulin into your bloodstream. In order to cope with the feeling of tiredness that this process engenders, you may have another sugar-containing 'food' or drink. And so the cycle repeats itself day after day through endless cups of sweet tea and coffee, and large numbers of chocolate bars, sweets and biscuits (laden with harmful trans fats). Eventually, in some people the body can no longer cope and they start to develop diabetes mellitus.

If you feel peckish in between your three main meals of the day (and I do strongly recommend that you try to have three square meals daily), then try some of the following possibilities:

- Fresh fruit – bananas, apples, satsumas, pears, strawber ries, blackcurrants, peaches, melons, etc. are all nutritious and can involve next-to-no preparation time

- Dried fruits – dates, figs and currants are particularly good ways of obtaining extra energy and also contain many valuable minerals

- Freshly squeezed orange juice or freshly pressed apple or pineapple juice – you should avoid 'fruit juices' made with concentrates, and, of course, always avoid 'fruit drinks' that contain added sugar

- A glass of milk, with a honey sandwich (made with wholemeal bread and butter)

- A carton of natural yoghurt perhaps sweetened with some honey.

In the next section, I shall give you the ingredients of a good breakfast.

Cortisol

As I mentioned earlier in this book, high levels of the hormone cortisol circulating in the blood can inhibit the action of the enzyme delta-6-desaturase. This enzyme occurs twice in the diagram on page 50 (Figure 5). First, it is used to help convert the parent essential fatty acids linoleic acid and alpha-linolenic acid into their respective omega-6 and omega-3 fatty acid derivatives. Second, delta-6-desaturase is one of the enzymes that helps in the conversion of EPA into DHA. For the reasons explained in Chapter 5, you should avoid taking any DHA in supplements. This means that the DHA you need should be derived from EPA. So it is helpful to reduce the circulating levels of cortisol.

The levels of the steroid hormone cortisol rise in the blood as a result of stresses such as:

- Anxiety

- Fear

- Pain

- Infections

- Low blood sugar levels

- Haemorrhage (bleeding)

- Starvation.

So, to reduce the circulating cortisol levels, you should work on trying to reduce these factors in your life.

Try to learn to cope with circumstances that make you anxious or fearful. Exercise, and some of the complementary therapies mentioned below, should help here. You could also ask your doctor to refer you for cognitive behavioural therapy, or CBT for short, which is a short form of psychotherapy which some patients find helpful. (In cognitive behaviour-al therapy, the therapist helps correct the distorted thought patterns and low self-image from which the patient may suffer.)

You should certainly avoid pain. You should also try to ensure that you do not go without three well-balanced proper meals daily, so that your blood sugar levels do not drop during the day. Make time for a good nourishing breakfast each morning. My usual breakfast, which helps set me up for the long working day ahead consists of:

- Muesli (made without added sugar or salt) that is rich in dried fruits, nuts and seeds

- Honey to sweeten the muesli

- Full-cream whole fresh milk – sometimes I prepare the muesli the evening before by adding milk to a bowl of it and leaving it in the refrigerator overnight

- A glass of freshly squeezed orange juice

- Four VegEPA capsules – I take my other four capsules each evening.

Avoid allowing your body weight to become so low that your body interprets this as starvation and raises the levels of cortisol.

Exercise

As your sleep improves on VegEPA and your energy levels rise, you will find that you can cope with increasing levels of physical activity. Gentle exercise is an excellent stress-buster which will help you to consolidate your recovery and continue to improve further. Good forms of exercise include:

- Walking – particularly enjoyable if you have a friend or partner to accompany you

- Cycling – starting at a gentle comfortable speed

- Swimming.

In his excellent book *Living with M.E.: The Chronic/Post-viral Fatigue Syndrome*, Dr Charles Shepherd, who is a world authority on chronic fatigue syndrome and Medical Director to the M.E.

Association, recommends that patients with chronic fatigue syndrome should continue to enjoy sexual intercourse with their partners, or at least some form of physical intimacy. Further details appear in Chapter 15 of his book.

Depression

Many chronic fatigue syndrome patients often feel depressed. Sometimes this is because of the results of the chronic fatigue syndrome, such as an inability to work or a loss of self-esteem. Some patients have told me that they were not feeling depressed in spite of being told that depression (and not chronic fatigue syndrome) was the correct diagnosis repeatedly by their doctor; eventually, they gave in and thought that perhaps the doctor must be right after all. In fairness to their doctors, some of the clinical features of chronic fatigue syndrome are similar to those that can occur in depression. It is no surprise, then, that some patients may be told they are suffering from depression rather than chronic fatigue syndrome.

It is common for patients, whether they have a diagnosis of depression or chronic fatigue syndrome, to be prescribed SSRI (or SSRI-like) antidepressant drugs. The main SSRI and SSRI-like antidepressants include:

- Fluoxetine (Prozac)

- Paroxetine (Seroxat or Paxil)

- Sertraline (Lustral or Zoloft)

- Citalopram (Cipramil or Celexa)

- Fluvoxamine (Faverin or Luvox)

- Escitalopram (Cipralex)

- Venlafaxine (Efexor or Effexor)

- Reboxetine (Edronax)

- Mirtazapine (Zispin or Remeron)

- Nefazodone (Dutonin or Serzone).

In this list, the non-proprietary name has been given first, followed by one or more trade names in parentheses. Different trade names are often used in different countries. For instance, paroxetine is known as Seroxat in the United Kingdom, and as Paxil in the United States.

There are other classes of antidepressants in common use, such as the tricyclic antidepressants (for example, amitriptyline and clomipramine) and monoamine oxidase inhibitors.

Fortunately, pure EPA (that is DHA-free), in the dose recommended by me for chronic fatigue syndrome (see above), has been found to be an effective antidepressant. Details of the use of EPA as an antidepressant appear in the book co-authored by Hilary Boyd and me entitled *The Natural Way to Beat Depression: The Groundbreaking Discovery of EPA to Change your Life*, which was published in 2004. This book also gives details of different conventional antidepressants and how to come off antidepressant medication. The most important point to note is that you should never simply stop your antidepressant medication without medical advice and supervision. This is because of the adverse effects that can occur when coming off such medication. Stopping an SSRI-like drug, for example, should happen gradually, and under strict medical guidance.

Remember too that, in addition to EPA, there are other non-drug treatments that can help improve mood. One example is cognitive behavioural therapy or CBT for short, which has already been mentioned briefly (see page 122). If you would like cognitive behavioural therapy you should see your family doctor for a referral to a psychologist or psychiatrist with expertise in this therapy.

Complementary therapies

There are several types of complementary therapy that can help relax your muscles and act as stress-busters.

Massage therapy

There are various forms of massage therapy available. They are good ways of helping you to feel more relaxed and less stressed. In one form, Shiatsu, the practitioner will carry out a form of acupressure in which certain points in the body are especially stimulated, perhaps by the use of the thumbs, fingers, elbows or even knees.

Aromatherapy

Aromatherapy involves the massage of essential oils into the skin. Your aromatherapist will be able to choose the most appropriate essential oils for your particular symptoms. In addition, you might want to consider using essential oils to help you relax or sleep. For example, you could try putting one or two drops of lavender oil on your pillow case when you go to bed. Inhaling the vapour from this oil might help you to sleep better.

Reflexology

Reflexology is a therapy which focuses on the feet. Those who have experienced it tend to be full of praise for the benefits they feel.

Daoyin Tao

Daoyin Tao is a complementary therapy that combines elements of massage therapy and aromatherapy. It was formulated in the 1990s by Anna-Louise Haigh.

The Alexander Technique

If you can find a good teacher, then the Alexander Technique has much to commend it. It is a method of mind and body re-education which can help to reduce stress and muscular tension. It also acts at a deep, unconscious level, to enable personal growth to take place.

I have been informed that one teacher of the Alexander Technique, who has a strong interest in research into the benefits of this therapy, has found that the effects on patients with chronic fatigue syndrome include:

- Increased blood flow

- Increased vitality

- Improved mood

- Less hopelessness

- More 'self-propelling'.

A good introduction is to be found in the books *The Alexander Principle: How to Use Your Body without Stress* by Dr Wilfred Barlow and *Body Learning: An Introduction to the Alexander Technique* by Michael Gelb.

Glossary

AA: arachidonic acid – a long chain polyunsaturated fatty omega-6 fatty acid created from the GLA via DGLA or eaten in the diet. It is of vital importance as a building block for eicosanoids.

Adrenal glands: glands lying just above the kidneys. The outer part of the glands secrete the stress hormone cortisol. The adrenal glands are sometimes also called the suprarenal glands.

Adrenic acid: an omega-6 long-chain polyunsaturated fatty acid. It is formed from arachidonic acid.

ALA: alpha-linolenic acid – the essential (short chain) parent omega-3 fatty acid.

Alpha-linolenic acid: the essential (short chain) parent omega-3 fatty acid.

Amino acid: a building block of proteins.

Anhedonia: an inability, resulting from a disorder such as depression, to gain pleasure from activities that were previously found to be pleasurable.

Antibodies: special chemicals released by certain white blood cells (B lymphocytes). They bind to pathogenic organisms and their products. This allows pathogens to be identified by other white blood cells (phagocytes) which can then 'go in for the kill'.

Anticoagulant therapy: treatment (such as heparin, warfarin, acenocoumarol or phenindione) used to thin the blood.

Arachidonic acid: a long chain polyunsaturated fatty omega-6 fatty acid created from the GLA via DGLA or eaten in the diet. It is of vital importance as a building block for eicosanoids.

Atrial fibrillation: a pathological condition of the heart in which its upper two chambers ('atria') stop pumping properly.

Autoimmune response: an immune response against tissues of one's own body.

B cells: lymphocytes that produce antibodies.

Biotin: a B vitamin.

Carcinoid syndrome: a syndrome caused by carcinoid tumours. A patient may flush, suffer from diarrhoea, vomiting and stomach (abdominal) pains.

Cardiomyopathy: a pathological condition in which the heart is enlarged.

CDC: the Centers for Disease Control and Prevention in Atlanta, Georgia.

Choline: a molecule that forms a polar head group in phospholipids.

Cortisol: a steroid hormone produced by the outer part of the adrenal glands (the adrenal cortex). Its levels rise in the blood as a result of stresses such as anxiety, fear, pain, infections, low blood sugar levels, haemorrhage and starvation. It inhibits the enzyme delta-6-desaturase.

Delta-6-desaturase: an enzyme that has two important functions in the synthesis of fatty acids. First, it is used to help convert the parent essential fatty acids, linoleic acid and alpha-linolenic acid, into their respective omega-6 and omega-3 fatty acid derivatives, respectively. Second, delta-6-desaturase is one of the enzymes that helps in the conversion of EPA into DHA.

Deoxyribonucleic acid: also known as DNA. This is the main molecule of heredity, which carries genetic information through the generations.

DGLA: dihomo-gamma-linolenic acid – an omega-6 long chain polyunsaturated fatty acid that the body can convert into arachidonic acid. It is of vital importance as a building block for eicosanoids.

DHA: docosahexaenoic acid – an omega-3 long chain polyunsaturated fatty acid that can be made from EPA. It is important in maintaining the correct structure of cell membranes.

Dihomo-gamma-linolenic acid: an omega-6 long chain polyunsaturated fatty acid that the body can convert into arachidonic acid. It is of vital importance as a building block for eicosanoids.

DNA: Deoxyribonucleic acid - the main molecule of heredity, which carries genetic information through the generations.

Docosahexaenoic acid: an omega-3 long chain polyunsaturated fatty acid that can be made from EPA. It is important in maintaining the correct structure of cell membranes.

Double-blind clinical trial: a trial involving both an active putative treatment and a placebo in which both the patients and the doctors or researchers do not know who is taking the active treatment and who the placebo during the whole course of the actual trial.

DPA: docosapentaenoic acid. There are actually two forms of DPA. One is a long-chain polyunsaturated omega-6 fatty acid, while the other is a long-chain polyunsaturated omega-3 fatty acid.

DVT: deep-vein thrombosis, or 'economy class syndrome'. Clots form in the deep veins of the calf muscles during extended periods of inactivity. Its consequences can be life-threatening.

Eicosanoids: families of thromboxanes, prostaglandins, leukotrienes and hydroxy fatty acids. These are of importance in maintaining the health of cells and tissues.

Eicosapentaenoic acid: an omega-3 long chain polyunsaturated fatty acid that is of vital importance as a building block for eicosanoids, sleep mediators, and interferons. It is viricidal (kills viruses).

Embolism: usually refers to a clot occurring in a blood vessel when it should not do so.

Emotional lability: a mood that easily and readily swings between highs and lows.

Enzyme: a biological catalyst that helps chemical reactions to take place much faster.

EPA: eicosapentaenoic acid – an omega-3 long chain polyunsaturated fatty acid that is of vital importance as a building block for eicosanoids, sleep mediators, and interferons. It is viricidal (kills viruses).

Endocrine system: a system consisting of a number of hormone-secreting organs such as the pancreas and adrenal glands.

Essential fatty acids: the parent omega-3 and omega-6 fatty acids linoleic acid and alpha-linolenic acid.

Ethyl-EPA: an ethyl ester form of EPA that is ultra-pure. It is the form of EPA that has been used in many major research studies and is the form that biotechnology companies are trying to bring to the market for the treatment of illnesses such as depression, Huntington's disease and schizophrenia. It is also the form of pure EPA that is found in VegEPA.

Evening primrose oil: oil from the seeds of the evening primrose plant. It is rich in the omega-6 fatty acid GLA.

Fasciculation: fine movements of small regions of muscles.

Gamma-linoleic acid: an omega-6 long chain polyunsaturated fatty acid that the body can convert into DGLA.

GLA: gamma-linoleic acid – an omega-6 long chain polyunsaturated fatty acid that the body can convert into DGLA.

Highly unsaturated fatty acid: an unsaturated fatty acid containing several double bonds between carbon atoms. Examples are EPA and GLA.

Hormones: chemical substances produced by endocrine and other glands. They circulate in the blood and influence various bodily functions.

HUFA: a commonly used abbreviation for highly unsaturated fatty acid.

Hydrogenated fats: these are the result of artificial processes in which vegetable oils, which are liquid at room temperature, are turned into hardened solids that are rich in trans fats.

Hydroxy fatty acids: special derivatives of fatty acids that are needed for the well-being of the body.

Hyperthyroidism: a condition in which there is overactivity of the thyroid gland.

Hypothyroidism: a condition in which there is underactivity of the thyroid gland.

Interferons: natural chemicals made from EPA that are important in helping the body to fight against viral infections.

Ischaemic heart disease: a pathological condition in which the blood supply to the heart is compromised, for example following a heart attack.

Keshan disease: a disease probably caused by a deficiency of selenium in the diet, in which the heart muscle degenerates.

LA: linoleic acid – the essential (short chain) parent omega-6 fatty acid.

Leukotrienes: special derivatives of fatty acids (such as EPA) that are needed for the well-being of the body.

Linoleic acid: the essential (short chain) parent omega-6 fatty acid.

Lymphocytes: these are a type of white blood cell.

Magnetic resonance imaging: a form of scanning that uses magnetic fields and radiowaves. It can produce highly accurate images of the body.

M.E.: myalgic encephalomyelitis. Another name for chronic fatigue syndrome.

Micromole: A micromole is one millionth of a mole. So a micromole of carbon-12 has a mass of 12 micrograms.

Microgram: A unit of mass (weight). A microgram is one-millionth of a gram, and one-billionth of a kilogram.

Milligram: A unit of mass (weight). A milligram is one-thousandth of a gram, and one millionth of a kilogram. The scientific abbreviation for milligram is mg.

Mole: A mole is a scientific measure referring to the mass (weight) of a substance that contains a certain specified number of molecules (or atoms) of that substance. For example, one mole of the commonest form of the element carbon, known as carbon-12, has a mass of exactly 12 grams. The scientific abbreviation for mole is mol.

MRI: magnetic resonance imaging. A way of obtaining the detailed anatomical structure of the body.

MRS: magnetic resonance spectroscopy. A way of gleaning chemical information about the body.

Myalgia: muscle pain.

Neurotic disorders: psychiatric disorders such as phobias in which patients experience symptoms that are unpleasant and not in tune with their personalities.

Neurotransmitter: a chemical such as dopamine or serotonin that jumps across the gap between nerve cells, thereby allowing messages to pass from one nerve cell to another.

Niacin: a B vitamin.

NK cells: natural killer white blood cells that engage in NK cell activity.

NK cell activity: this is natural killer cell activity directed against cells that have become infected by viruses and also tumour cells. It is carried out by large granular lymphocytes that recognize these cells.

Omega-3 fatty acids: a family of fatty acids that includes alpha-linolenic acid, EPA and DHA.

Omega-6 fatty acids: a family of fatty acids that includes linoleic acid, GLA, dihomo-gamma-linolenic acid and arachidonic acid.

Phaeochromocytoma: a tumour that secretes adrenaline-like hormones. They are rare tumours, and when they do occur they are often found in the adrenal glands.

Phospholipid: a complex molecule found in all cell membranes that include fatty acids.

Placebo: an inactive or 'dummy' substance that looks identical to the active treatment in a double-blind trial.

Polyunsaturated fatty acid: an unsaturated fatty acid containing at least one double bond between carbon atoms. Examples are EPA and GLA.

Prostaglandins: important families of substances formed from fatty acids such as EPA that are essential for the well-being of the body.

Protozoa: single-celled animals such as Amoebae.

PUFA: a commonly used abbreviation for polyunsaturated fatty acid.

Pulmonary embolism: clots in blood vessels of the lungs that can prove to be fatal.

Scurvy: a disorder that occurs in vitamin C deficiency that can present with bleeding gums and skin problems.

SSRIs: a class of antidepressant drugs that are selective serotonin re-uptake inhibitors. They increase the amount of the neurotransmitter serotonin in the gaps between nerve cells in the brain. Examples include fluoxetine, citalopram, escitalopram, fluvoxamine, paroxetine and sertraline.

T cells: these are types of lymphocytes.

Tc cells: these are T-cytotoxic cells. They destroy infected cells.

Th1 cells: these are type-1 helper T cells. They help other white blood cells to engulf and destroy pathogens (disease causing organisms).

Th2 cells: these are type-2 helper T cells. They help B cells to reproduce and to make antibodies.

Thromboxanes: special derivatives of fatty acids that are needed for the well-being of the body.

Trace elements: mineral elements that are needed in the diet in trace amounts.

Trans fats: the artificial trans fats are created in the industrial process of manufacturing hydrogenated fats. They have deleterious effects on cell membranes.

Trans fatty acids: another name for trans fats.

Triterpines: naturally occurring molecules that have several health-giving properties. They are found in virgin evening primrose oil.

Unsaturated fatty acids: fatty acids in which one or more carbon double bonds occur in each molecule.

Ventricles: chambers in the brain or heart, each of which has two ventricles.

Virgin evening primrose oil: evening primrose oil that is cold-pressed and non-raffinated so that it retains much of its goodness, including the presence of triterpines.

References

Afari, N. and Buchwald, D. (2003). Chronic fatigue syndrome: a review. *American Journal of Psychiatry* **160**: 221-236.

American Heart Association (1996). AHA Scientific Statement: Fish Consumption, Fish Oil, Omega-3 Fatty Acids and Cardiovascular Disease, #71-0241. *Circulation* **106**: 2747-2757.

American Psychiatric Association (2000). *Diagnostic and Statistical Manual of Mental Disorders*, Fourth edition, Text Revision (DSM-IV-TR). Washington D.C.: American Psychiatric Association.

Barlow, W. (2001). *The Alexander Principle: How to Use Your Body without Stress*. London: Orion.

Beard, G. (1869). Neurasthenia, or nervous exhaustion. *Boston Medical and Surgical Journal* **3**: 217-221.

Behan, P.O., Behan, W.M.H. and Horrobin, D. (1990). Effect of high doses of essential fatty acids on the postviral fatigue syndrome. *Acta Neurologica Scandinavica* **82**: 209-216.

Carrasco, L. (1995). Modification of membrane permeability by animal viruses. In: K. Maramorosch, F.A. Murphy and A.J. Shatkin (editors) *Advances in Virus Research*, **Volume 45**. Academic Press: New York, pp. 61-112.

Caligiuri, M., Murray, C., Buchwald, D., Levine, H., Cheney, P., Peterson, D., Komaroff, A.L. and Ritz, J. (1987). Phenotypic and functional deficiency of natural killer cells in patients with chronic fatigue syndrome. *Journal of Immunology* **139**: 3306-3313.

Chaudhuri, A., Condon, B.R., Gow, J.W., Brennan, D. and Hadley, D.M. (2003). Proton magnetic resonance spectroscopy of basal ganglia in chronic fatigue syndrome. *Neuroreport* **14**: 225-228.

Dale, R.C., Church, A.J., Surtees, R.A., Lees, A.J., Adcock, J.E., Harding, B., Neville, B.G. and Giovannoni, G. (2004). Encephalitis lethargica syndrome: 20 new cases and evidence of basal ganglia autoimmunity. *Brain* **127**: 21-33.

De Vriese, S.R., Christophe, A.B. and Maes, M. (2004). In humans, the seasonal variation in poly-unsaturated fatty acids is related to the seasonal variation in violent suicide and serotonergic markers of violent suicide. *Prostaglandins Leukotrienes and Essential Fatty Acids* **71**: 13-18.

Deale, H. and Adams, S. (1894). Neurasthenia in young women. *American Journal of Obstetrics* **29**: 190-195.

Editorial (1970). Epidemic malaise. *British Medical Journal* **1**: 1-2.

Editorial. (1956). A new clinical entity? *Lancet* **270**: 789-790.

Farmer, A., Fowler, T., Scourfield, J. and Thapar, A. (2004). Prevalence of chronic disabling fatigue in children and adolescents. *British Journal of Psychiatry* **184**: 477-481.

Fekety, R. (1994). Infection and chronic fatigue syndrome. In: S. Straus (editor) *Chronic Fatigue Syndrome*. New York, USA: Marcel Dekker.

Freeman, C.P.L. (1998). Neurotic disorders. In: Johnstone, E.C., Freeman, C.P.L. and Zealley, A.K. (editors) *Companion to Psychiatric Studies*, 6th edition. Edinburgh: Churchill Livingstone.

Fukuda, K., Straus, S.E., Hickie, I., Sharpe, M.C., Dobbins, J.G., Komaroff, A.L. and the International Chronic Fatigue Syndrome Study Group (1994). The Chronic Fatigue Syndrome: A Comprehensive Approach to its Definition and Study. *Annals of Internal Medicine* **121**: 953-959.

Gelb, M.J. (2004). *Body Learning: An Introduction to the Alexander Technique*. London: Aurum Press.

Graham, J. (1984). *Evening Primrose Oil: Its Remarkable Properties and its Use in the Treatment of a Wide Range of Conditions*. Wellingborough, Northamptonshire, U.K.: Thorsons Publishers Ltd.

Hamburger, M., Riese, U., Graf, H., Melzig, M.F., Ciesielski, S., Baumann, D., Dittmann, K. and Wegner, C. (2002). Constituents in evening primrose oil with radical scavenging, cyclooxygenase, and neutrophil elastase inhibitory activities. *Journal of Agricultural and Food Chemistry* **50**: 5533-5538

Hibbeln, J.R. (1998). Fish consumption and major depression [letter]. *Lancet* **351**: 1213.

Hooper, R (2005). Chronic fatigue syndrome is not all in the mind. *New Scientist* **2509**: 9.

Jones, J.F., Nisenbaum, R., Solomon, L., Reyes, M. and Reeves, W.C. (2004). Chronic fatigue syndrome and other fatiguing illnesses in adolescents: a population-based study. *Journal of Adolescent Health* **35**: 34-40.

Kaushik, N., Fear, D., Richards, S.C., McDermott, C.R., Nuwaysir, E.F., Kellam, P., Harrison, T.J., Tyrrell, D.A., Holgate, S.T. and Kerr, J.R. Gene expression in peripheral blood mononuclear cells from patients with chronic fatigue syndrome. *Journal of Clinical Pathology* **58**:826-832.

J.R. Klimas, N.G., Salvato, F.R., Morgan, R. and Fletcher, M.A. (1990). Immunologic abnormalities in chronic fatigue syndrome. *Journal of Clinical Microbiology* **28**: 1403-1410.

Maes, M., Cosyns, P., Meltzer, H.Y., De Meyer, F. and Peeters, D. (1993). Seasonality in violent suicide but not in nonviolent suicide or homicide. *American Journal of Psychiatry* **150**: 1380-1385.

McEvedy, C.P., Griffiths, A., and Hall, T. (1966) *British Medical Journal* **2**, 1300.

McEvedy, C.P. and Beard, A.W. (1970). Royal Free Epidemic of 1955:

a reconsideration. *British Medical Journal* **1**: 7-11.

Mozaffarian, D., Psaty, B.M., Rimm, E.B., Lemaitre, R.N., Burke, G.L., Lyles, M.F., Lefkowitz, D. and Siscovick, D.S. (2004). Fish intake and risk of incident atrial fibrillation. *Circulation* **110**: 368-373.

Nemets, B., Stahl, Z. and Belmaker, R.H. (2002). Addition of omega-3 fatty acid to maintenance medication treatment for recurrent unipolar depressive disorder. *American Journal of Psychiatry* **159**: 477-479.

Puri, B.K. (2004). The use of eicosapentaenoic acid in the treatment of chronic fatigue syndrome. *Prostaglandins, Leukotrienes and Essential Fatty Acids* **70**: 399-401.

Puri, B.K. (2004). Monomodal rigid-body registration and applications to the investigation of the effects of eicosapentaenoic acid intervention in neuropsychiatric disorders. *Prostaglandins, Leukotrienes and Essential Fatty Acids* **71**: 177-179.

Puri, B.K. (2004). The clinical advantages of cold-pressed non-raffinated evening primrose oil over refined preparations. *Medical Hypotheses* **62**: 116-118.

Puri, B.K. and Boyd, H. (2004). *The Natural Way to Beat Depression: The Groundbreaking Discovery of EPA to Change your Life*. London: Hodder and Stoughton.

Puri, B.K. (2004/5). Lipids, eicosapentaenoic acid, and depression. In: Mostofsky, D.I., and Yehuda, S. (editors) *Nutrients, Stress, Medical Disorders*. New Jersey, USA: Humana Press.

Puri, B.K., Counsell, S.J., Hamilton, G., Richardson, A.J. and Horrobin, D.F. (2001). Eicosapentaenoic acid in treatment-resistant depression associated with symptom remission, structural brain changes and reduced neuronal phospholipid turnover. *International Journal of Clinical Practice* **55**: 560-563.

Puri, B.K., Counsell, S.J., Richardson, A.J. and Horrobin, D.F. (2002). Eicosapentaenoic acid in treatment-resistant depression. *Archives of General Psychiatry* **59**: 91-92.

Puri, B.K., Counsell, S.J., Zaman, R., Main, J., Collins, A.J., Hajnal, J.V. and Davey, N.J. (2002). Relative increase in choline in the occipital cortex in chronic fatigue syndrome. *Acta Psychiatrica Scandinavica* **106**: 224-226.

Puri, B.K., Holmes, J. and Hamilton, G. (2004). Eicosapentaenoic acid-rich essential fatty acid supplementation in chronic fatigue syndrome associated with symptom remission and structural brain changes. *International Journal of Clinical Practice* 58: 297-299.

Ruiz-Cabello, J. and Cohen, J.S. (1992). Phospholipid metabolites as indicators of cancer cell function. *NMR in Biomedicine* **5**: 226-233.

Sacks, O. (1987). *Awakenings*. New Jersey: Simon & Schuster.

Shepherd, C. (1999). *Living with M.E.: The Chronic/Post-viral Fatigue Syndrome*. London: Vermilion.

Singleton, N., Bumpstead, R., O'Brien, M., Lee, A. and Meltzer, H. (2000). *Psychiatric Morbidity among Adults living in Private Households, 2000: Summary Report*. London: Office for National Statistics.

Skowera, A., Cleare, A., Blair, D., Bevis, L., Wessely, S.C. and Peakman, M. (2004). High levels of type 2 cytokine-producing cells in chronic fatigue syndrome. *Clinical and Experimental Immunology* **135**: 294-302.

Thorlaksdottir, A.Y., Skuladottir, G.V., Tryggvadottir, L., Stefansdottir, S., Hafsteinsdottir, H., Ogmundsdottir, H.O., Eyfjord, J.E., Jonsson, J.J. and Hardardottir, I. (2004). Positive association between DNA strand breaks in peripheral blood mononuclear cells and polyunsaturated fatty acids in red blood cells. *Abstracts of the Sixth Congress of the International Society for the Study of Fatty Acids and Lipids Poster* (4-5), page 129.

Tirelli, V., Pinto, A., Marotta, G., Crovato, M., Quaia, M., De Paoli, P., Galligioni, E. and Santini, G. (1993). Clinical and immunologic study of 205 patients with chronic fatigue syndrome: a case series from Italy. *Archives of Internal Medicine* **153**: 116-120.

Tomoda, A., Miike, T., Yamada, E., Honda, H., Moroi, T., Ogawa, M.,

Ohtani, Y. and Morishita, S. (2000). Chronic fatigue syndrome in childhood. *Brain and Development* **22**: 60-64.

Van Deusen, E. (1869). Observations of a form of nervous prostration, (neurasthenia), culminating in insanity. *American Journal of Insanity* 445-461.

Visser, J., Blauw, B., Hinloopen, B., Brommer, E., de Kloet, E.R., Kluft, C. and Nagelkerken, L. (1998). CD4 T lymphocytes from patients with chronic fatigue syndrome have decreased interferon-gamma production and increased sensitivity to dexamethasone. *Journal of Infectious Diseases* **177**: 451-454.

Warren, G., McKendrick, M. and Peet, M. (1999). The role of essential fatty acids in chronic fatigue syndrome. *Acta Neurologica Scandinavica* **99**: 112-116.

World Health Organization (1992). *The ICD-10 Classification of Mental and Behavioural Disorders*. Geneva: World Health Organization.

Young, D.A.B. (1995). Florence Nightingale's fever. *British Medical Journal* **311**: 1697-1700.

Further sources of information

Recommended books

Shepherd, C. (1999). *Living with M.E.: The Chronic/Post-viral Fatigue Syndrome*. London: Vermilion.
    This is an excellent guide to all aspects of living with chronic fatigue syndrome. Simply the best book on this subject and very comprehensive. The author, Dr Charles Shepherd, speaks from personal experience, having suffered from chronic fatigue syndrome and manages to convey large amounts of up-to-date research information in a way that is easy to read and understand.

Barlow, W. (2001).*The Alexander Principle: How to Use Your Body without Stress*. London: Orion.

Gelb, M.J. (2004). *Body Learning: An Introduction to the Alexander Technique*. London: Aurum Press.

Graham, J. (1984). *Evening Primrose Oil: Its Remarkable Properties and its Use in the Treatment of a Wide Range of Conditions*. Wellingborough, Northamptonshire, U.K.: Thorsons Publishers Ltd.

Puri, B.K. and Boyd, H. (2004). *The Natural Way to Beat Depression: The Groundbreaking Discovery of EPA to Change your Life*. London: Hodder and Stoughton.

Internet web sites

Daoyin Tao® International

Useful information about this complementary therapy.
www.daoyintao.com

Google

Typing in chronic fatigue syndrome or M.E. into the Google search engine will furnish you with some of the latest work in this area.
www.google.com

ME Association

This is a very useful site with listings of local societies throughout the world.
www.meassociation.org.uk

PubMed

This allows you access to the abstracts of all recent medical and scientific research publications from international journals, without charge. Just type in the name of the authors (surname and then initial) and/or the subject area.
www.ncbi.nim.nih.gov/PubMed

VegEPA

This is a good site for research and information about fatty acids and diseases such as chronic fatigue syndrome/M.E. It also has information about VegEPA. The product ordering line is 00 44 845 1300 424 from outside the UK, and 0845 1300 424 from within the UK.
www.vegepa.com

Useful names and addresses

Action for M.E.
P O Box 1302
Wells
Somerset
BA5 1YE
UK
Tel: 01749 670799

ANZMES
P O Box 36 307
Northcote
Auckland 1309
New Zealand

Australia – there are M.E./CFS Societies for the Australian Capital Territory, New South Wales, Northern Territory, Queensland, South Australia and the Northern Territory, Victoria and Tasmania, and Western Australia. Full details are available via the internet.

CFIDS Association
P O Box 220398
Charlotte
NC 28222-0389
USA
Tel: 00 1 800 442 3437 (toll free in the USA)

Daoyin Tao® International
15 Montpellier Parade
Harrogate
North Yorkshire
England
UK
HG1 2TG
Tel: ++44 (0) 1423 567766

Irish M.E. Support Group
P O Box 3075
Dublin 2
Tel: (01) 235 0965

MEASA (M.E. Association of South Africa)
P O Box 1802
Umhlanga Rocks
4320
Kwa Zulu Natal
South Africa

The National CFIDS Foundation
103 Aletha Road
Needham
MA 02192
USA
Tel: 00 1 781 449 3535

M.E. Association
4 Corringham Road
Stanford le Hope
Essex SS17 0AH
UK
Tel: 01375 642466

M.E. Canada
246 Queen Street
Suite 400
Ottawa
Ontario
K1P 5E4
Canada
Tel: (613) 563 7514

VegEPA, VegeCO and mini VegeCO manufacturer:
Igennus Ltd.
St John's Innovation Centre
Cowley Road
Cambridge CB4 0WS
England, UK
Tel: 00 44 845 1300 424 from outside the UK, and 0845 1300 424
(low cost) from within the UK

Index

A

AA - see arachidonic acid
acrylamide, 120
acupressure, 126
Adams, 10
ADHD - see attention-deficit
    hyperactivity disorder
adrenal gland, 91
adrenaline, 91
adrenic acid, 33, 35
Afar, Niloofar, 20
alcohol, 95, 116
alcoholism, 90, 95, 112
Alexander technique, 127
alpha-linolenic acid, 49, 50, 51,
    83
    laboratory reference range,
    114
anaemia, 87, 88, 89, 93
Anchor Butter, 120
animal husbandry, 99
antibodies, 26, 29
antidepressants, 91, 124-125
anti-egg white injury factor, 91
arachidonic acid, 33, 35, 49, 50,
    51, 57, 75
    laboratory reference range,
    114

arcus senilis, 101
aromatherapy, 126
arthritis, 77, 102, 105
ascorbate - see vitamin C
ascorbic acid - see vitamin C
atrial fibrillation, 104-105, 120
attention-deficit hyperactivity
    disorder
    improvement, 101
    treatment with EPA, 80
autoimmune response, 30
avidin, 91

B

B cells, 28, 29
Barlow, Wilfred, 127, 142
basal ganglia, 42, 43
Beard, Alfred William, 9, 15, 16,
    22
Beard, George, 12
Behan, Peter, 31-35, 37, 56, 58,
    63
Behan, Wilhelmina, 31-33,
    56, 58, 63
Bell, Jimmy, 42
beta-oxidation, 84

biotin, 85, 86, 91-92
blood clotting, 102-104
bowel cancer, reducing the risk
of, 97
Boyd, Hilary, 125, 142
brain
anatomy, 42
biochemistry, 36-44
change in size following fatty
acids, 69
cortex, 41
fog, 7
grey matter, 41
hemisphere, 68
lateral ventricles, 68
white matter, 41
breasts, painful, 75
Bruce, Dr David, 11
brucellosis, 11
Browning, Elizabeth Barrett, 10-11
Buchwald, Dedra, 20
Burkitt's lymphoma, 111
butter, 119, 120
Bydder, Graeme, 68

C

cadmium, 77, 78
caffeine, 116
Candida albicans, 111
canola oil , 117
carcinogenesis, 82
carcinoid syndrome, 90-91
carcinoid tumour, 90-91
cardiomyopathy, 94
CBT - see cognitive behavioural
therapy
CDC - see Centers for Disease

Control and Prevention
cell, 46
cell membrane, 46, 51
Centers for Disease Control and
Prevention, 16, 111-112
revised diagnostic criteria,
16-18
cerebrospinal fluid, 14, 68
CFIDS - see chronic fatigue and
immune dysfunction
Chaudhuri, Abhijit, 43-44
chicken pox, 23
chlorophyll, 94
choline, 41-44, 47, 55
chronic fatigue and immune
dysfunction, 19
cobalamins, 87
cobalt, 87
cod liver oil, disadvantages of,
78-79
coenzyme R - see biotin
cofactors, 84-86
coffee, 116
cognitive behavioural therapy,
122, 125
cola, 116
Collins, Alan, 41
commensals, 27
complementary therapies,
126-127
concentration
impairment, 18, 22, 55
improvement, 37, 100-101
copper, 93
corn oil, 118
cortisol, 116, 121-123
cottonseed oil, 118
Counsell, Serena, 41
COX, 53

Cox, Jane, 42-43
cyclo-oxygenase, 53, 85
creatine, 41
cyanocobalamin, 87

D

Dale, Russell, 25
Daoyin Tao, 126, 143
Davey, Nick, 41
Deale, 10
deep vein thrombosis, 102-103
delta-5-desaturase, 84
delta-6-desaturase, 50, 51, 56-
    57, 75, 83, 84, 122
    effect of cortisol on, 116
    effect of manufactured trans
        fats on, 119
    effect of virus infections on,
        54
deoxyribonucleic acid - see DNA
depression, 36, 42, 124-125
    treatment with EPA, 80, 98-
        99
dermatitis, 89, 90
DGLA, 49, 50, 51, 57, 75
    laboratory reference range,
        114
DHA, 33, 50, 51, 79-82
diabetes mellitus, 75, 102, 121
dibenzofurans, 77
dietary fibre, 97
dihomo-gamma-linolenic acid -
    see DGLA
dioxins, 77
DNA, 23, 46
    damage by DHA, 81
    damage by linoleic acid, 81
Dobbins, James G., 16-18

docosahexaenoic acid - see DHA
docosapentaenoic acid, 84
DPA, 33
DSM-IV-TR, 12-13
DVT, 102-103

E

eczema, 102
Efamol, 75
Efamol Ltd, 75
Efamaol Marine, 60, 65, 66
eggs, raw, 91-92
eicosanoids, 52, 75, 100
eicosapentaenoic acid - see EPA
electrocardiogram, 104
elongase, 84
emotional lability, 14
encephalitis lethargica, 24-25
encephalomyelitis, 19
energy improvement, 100
enteroviruses, 111
enzyme, 50-51, 84-85
EPA, 24, 33, 36, 50, 51, 53, 57,
    80, 82, 85
    ethyl, 99
    laboratory reference range,
        114
    seasonal variation in, 98-99
epinephrine - see adrenaline
Epogam, 60-61
Epstein-Barr virus, 27, 53, 111
Eskimo diet, 101-102
ethyl EPA, 99
evening primrose oil, 74
    as a source of GLA, 57
    benefits, 75
    virgin, 57, 76-77
examination, physical, 110

exercise, 123-124
  malaise following, 18
  to counter stress, 116
eye q, 67

F

Farmer, Anne, 21
fasciculation, 14, 18
fatigue, 18, 23
fatty acids, 32-33, 35, 36, 46-73
Fekety, Robert, 11
fish, 49, 77-78
  pollutants in, 77-78
fish oil, disadvantages of, 78-79
flaxseed oil, 82
  why a very poor source of
    EPA, 83
flushes, hot, 94
folacin - see folic acid
folate - see folic acid
folic acid, 85, 86-87
free radicals, 81
Freeman, Christopher, 15
frying, 118, 120
Fukuda, Keiji, 16-18

G

gamma-linolenic acid - see GLA
Gelb, Michael, 127, 142
genetic information, 23
GLA, 33, 49, 50, 57, 75
  laboratory reference range,
    114
glandular fever, 27, 111
Graham, Judy, 75, 142
grapeseed oil, 118

H

Haigh, Anna-Louise, 126
hair
  follicles, 92
  improvement, 106
Hajnal, Joseph, 41, 68
Hamburger, Matthias, 76-77
Hamilton, Gavin, 66
headache, 18
heart disease, 101-105
helium, 38-39
herpesvirus, 111
Hibbeln, Joe, 98
Hickie, Ian, 16-18
highly unsaturated fatty acids,
    definition, 51
history, clinical, 109
Holmes, Joanne, 66
Horrobin, David, 31-33, 56, 58,
    63, 75, 101
household shortening, 118
HUFAs, definition, 51
Huntington's disease, 42
hydralazine, 89
hydrogenated vegetable fat, 119
hydrogenation, 119
hydroxocobalamin, 87
hydroxy fatty acids, 52
hysteria, 9, 45
  mass, 15-16
  epidemic, 15-16

I

ICD-10, 13, 18
immune system changes, 26-30
influenza, 23
  pandemic, 24-25
insulin, 121

interferons, 53, 85
International Chronic Fatigue
    Syndrome Study Group,
    16-18
Inuit, 101-102
investigations, laboratory, 110-111
iron, 93
isoniazid, 89, 90

J
Janssen, Pierre, 39
joint pain, 18, 102, 105

K
Kerr, Jonathan, 45
Keshan disease, 94
kidney stone, 92, 96
Komaroff, Anthony L., 16-18

L
lard, 118
large granular lymphocytes,
    28-30
lavender oil, 126
LC-PUFAs, definition, 51
lead, 77, 78
leukotrienes, 52
linoleic acid, 33, 49, 50, 51, 81-
    82
    content in oils, 117-118
    effect on delta-6-desaturase,
        117
    laboratory reference range, 114
lipo-oxygenase, 53, 85
liver
    enlargement, 14

detoxification, role in, 78
oils, disadvantages of, 78-79
Lockyer, Joseph, 39
long-chain polyunsaturated fatty
    acids, definition, 51
Los Angeles County Hospital,
    13-14, 24
LOX, 53
lumbar puncture, 68
lymphadenopathy, 14
lymph node tenderness, 18
lymphocytes, 28-29
    changes in chronic fatigue
        syndrome, 29-30
lysozyme, 27

M
macrocytic anaemia, 87, 88
Maes, Michael, 98
magnesium, 85, 94-95
Main, Janice, 41
maize-rich diet, 90
malabsorption, 86
Malta fever, 11
Manku, Mehar, 31-32, 38
massage therapy, 126
mastalgia, 75
mayonnaise, 118
McEvedy, Colin, 9, 15, 16, 22
M.E. - see myalgic
    encephalomyelitis
medical assessment, 108-112
Mediterranean fever, 11
megaloblastic anaemia, 87, 88
memory impairment, 18, 55
menopause, 94
mental state examination, 109
mercury, 77, 78

microbes, 25, 26-28, 87-88
micro-organisms - see microbes
mini VegeCO, 118, 146
mitochondria, 46
monoamine oxidase inhibitors, 125
Montgomery and Åsberg
        Depression Rating Scale,
        66, 67
mood improvement, 37, 98-99
Morse-Fisher, Nancy, 31-32, 38
Mozaffarian, Dariush, 104-105,
        120
MRI scanning, 38-41
multimineral supplements, 96
muscle features, 18, 22
mustard oil, 117
mutation, 81
myalgia, 14, 18
myalgic encephalomyelitis, 18-19

N

nails, improvement, 75, 106-107
narcolepsy, 112
neurasthenia, 10-13, 18
neuropathy, 102
neurospectroscopy, 38-44, 55
neurotic disorder, 13
niacin, 85, 86, 89-91
niacytin, 90
nicotine, 116
nicotinic acid - see niacin
Nightingale, Florence, 11
NK cells, 28-30
noradrenaline, 91
norepinephrine - see
        noradrenaline
nuclear envelope, 46
nucleus, 46

O

occipital cortex, 41, 42
octadecatetraenoic acid, 83
Oenothera biennis, 61, 74
olive oil, virgin, 118
omega-3, 32, 33, 37, 42, 48-54
omega-6, 32, 33, 35, 37, 42, 48,
        49-54
organelle, 46
organic lesions, 11
osteoarthritis - see arthritis
Oxford criteria, 36, 64

P

palm oil, 118
Pauling, Linus, 92
PCBs, 77, 78
peanut oil, 118
Peet, Malcolm, 35-36, 56, 63, 64
pellagra, 90
penicillamine, 89
phaeochromocytoma, 90, 91
phospholipases, 55
phospholipids, 46-47, 70
        breakdown by viruses, 55
placebo effect, 8
PMS - see premenstrual
        syndrome
PMT - see premenstrual
        tension
poliomyelitis, 14
polychlorinated biphenyls,
        77, 78
polychlorinated dibenzo-p-
        dioxins, 77
post-viral fatigue syndrome, 19,
        31, 58, 63
premenstrual syndrome, 75

premenstrual tension - see
        premenstrual syndrome
prostaglandins, 52
protein, 89
    deficiency, 90
Proust, Marcel, 11
psychosomatic illness, 9, 12, 16,
        22, 45
pulmonary embolism, 102-103
Puri, Basant, 41, 66, 69, 99, 125
PVFS - see post-viral fatigue
        syndrome
pyridoxal, 88
pyridoxamine, 89
pyridoxine, 88

R
Ramsay, William, 39
reading improvement, 101
red blood cell, 46
    fatty acids, 32-33, 35, 36,
        114
    studies, 36-37, 38
reflexology, 126
retroviruses, 111
rheumatoid arthritis - see
        arthritis
RNA, 23
Royal Free disease - see Royal
        Free Hospital outbreak
Royal Free Hospital outbreak, 9,
        14-16, 22, 24

S
Sacks, Oliver, 24
Saeed, Nadeem, 69
safflower oil, 118

scurvy, 93
selective serotonin re-uptake
        inhibitor - see SSRI
selenium, 85, 94
serotonin, 91
sesame oil, 118
Sharpe, Michael C., 16-18
Shepherd, Charles, 123-124, 142
Shiatsu, 126
shingles, 23
signs, 12
Sinclair, Hugh, 101-102
Singleton, Nicola, 20
skin improvement, 72, 75, 92,
        106
sleep, 18, 53, 100
    apnoea, 112
smoking, 116
sore throat, 18, 25-26
soyabean oil, 117
soybean lecithin oil, 118
soybean oil, 117
spectroscopy, 38-44
SSRI, 91, 124-125
starflower oil, 57
statistical significance, 32, 34-35
Straus, Stephen E., 16-18
Streptococcus, 25-26
stress, 115-116
    hormones, 116
subacute combined degeneration
        of the spinal cord, 88
sub-clinical infection, 23
sunflower oil, 118
sugar, 120-121
symptoms, 12
synovial fluid, 105

T

T cells, 28-30
Tc cells, 29
T-cytotoxic cells - see Tc cells
tea, 116
tetracosapentaenoic acid, 84
tetrahexaenoic acid, 84
Th1 cells, 29, 30
Th2 cells, 29, 30
Thorlaksdottir, 80-81, 82
thrombotic stroke, 102, 103
thromboxanes, 52
Tomoda, Akemi, 44
trace element, 93-95
trans fats, 119-121
tricyclic antidepressants, 125
triterpines, 77, 83
tryptophan, 89-90
type-1 helper cells - see Th1 cells
type-2 helper cells - see Th2 cells
type 2 immune response, 30

U

undulant fever, 11

V

Van Deusen, 12
VegeCO, 117-118, 146
VegEPA, 7, 8, 37, 71, 81, 143
    composition, 83
    DHA-free, 80
    dosage, 115
    enhancement of white blood
        cell functions, 77
    ethyl EPA in, 99
    free radical mopping up by,
        77
    freedom from vitamin A, 79
    triterpines in, 77
    ultra-pure EPA in, 80,
        81, 99
    virgin evening primrose oil
        in, 76
ventricles, brain, 68
    changes after fatty acid
        treatment, 69
viral infections, 22-26
    effects of EPA on, 53
    effects on fatty acids, 53-55
vitamin A
    dangers of, 79
    in fish oil, 78
    liver storage, 78
vitamin B_3 - see niacin
vitamin B_6, 85, 86, 88-89
vitamin B_{12}, 85, 86, 87-88
vitamin C, 85, 92-93
vitamin E, 60
vitamin H - see biotin
vitamin supplements, 95-96
von Economo encephalitis, 24-25

W

walnut oil, 117
weight, 105-106
wheat germ oil, 118
white matter, 42, 44
white blood cells, 26, 28-30, 46,
    77
white sugar, 50-51, 120-121
World Health Organization, 13
wound healing, 93

Y
Young, 11
yuppie 'flu, 19

Z
Zaman, Rashid, 41
zinc, 85, 93-94

Notes

Other Hammersmith Press titles from the same author

Attention Deficit Hyperactivity Disorder
a natural way to treat ADHD
Professor Basant K. Puri
160pp £14.99
ISBN: 1-905140-01-0
Published September 2005

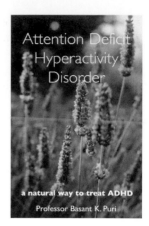

A fresh look at ADHD, the controversial condition that is being increasingly diagnosed in children in the developed world and treated with powerful drugs. Professor Basant Puri examines the underlying metabolic problems and dietary imbalances that may lie behind hyperactive behaviour, and the ways in which these deficiencies can be addressed. Parents and carers of children with ADHD will find new hope in combating this relentless condition.

Natural Energy
Professor Basant K. Puri
224 pp £14.99
ISBN: 1-905140-02-9
Due for publication: February 2007

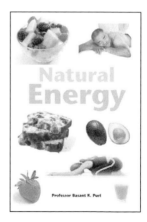

Extending the principles of treating M.E. and ADHD with a diet rich in phospho-lipids to the promotion of greater energy in any individual. Modern lifestyles are blamed for increasing tiredness experienced by the general population but poor diet has a much more significant role to play and there are clear ways to combat this trend and increase personal energy levels.

Other Hammersmith Press titles, continued

The Natural Energy Cookbook
Professor Basant K. Puri
224 pp   £14.99
ISBN: 1-905140-03-7
Due for publication: March 2007

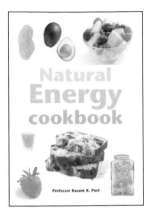

The practical way to achieve a diet high in phospho-lipids that is also delicious, varied and easy to prepare. Grouped around key ingredients, the book presents tried-and-tested recipes together with weekly menu plans.

About the author

Professor Basant K. Puri
MA (Cantab), PhD, MB, BChir, BSc (hons) MathSci, MRCPsych, DipStat, MMath

Dr Puri is Professor and Consultant at the MRI Unit, Imaging Sciences Department, MRC Clinical Sciences Centre, Hammersmith Hospital, London and Head of the Lipid Neuroscience Group, Imperial College, London.

Since the start of the new millennium, Professor Puri has been using natural fatty acids to treat patients with chronic fatigue syndrome. He has also been actively researching this disorder with colleagues at Imperial College London, using state-of-the-art electrophysiological and brain scanning techniques. His treatment approach and research findings have been described in authoritative medical journals and in lectures at international medical conferences.